Labor Relations in the Health Professions

William B. Werther, Jr., Ph.D.
Arbitrator, National Labor Panel,
American Arbitration Association;
Associate Professor of Management,
College of Business Administration,
Arizona State University,
Tempe, Arizona

Carol Ann Lockhart, R.N., M.S.
Chief, Office of Local Health Services,
Arizona Department of Health Services,
Phoenix, Arizona;
Instructor, College of Nursing,
Arizona State University,
Tempe, Arizona

Forewords by

Stephen M. Morris, M.H.A.
President, Samaritan Health Service,
Phoenix, Arizona;
Former President, American Hospital Association

Rosamond C. Gabrielson, R.N., M.A.
President, American Nurses' Association;
Consultant, Nursing Services,
Samaritan Health Service,
Phoenix, Arizona

Little, Brown and Company   Boston

• *Labor Relations in the Health Professions*

The Basis of Power – The Means of Change

Foreword

The need for a book explaining the basics of how to deal with a new
era in labor relations was apparent the moment the Taft-Hartley exemption was lifted from nonprofit hospitals. The law requires a new
awareness on the part of hospital administrators of what they can and
cannot do, and should and should not do, in the field of employee
relations. The law also clearly defines rights and restraints for hospital
employees in their dealings with grievances and management negotiations. Intrinsic to this new relationship between employees and administrators is the responsibility of both to maintain the interests of
the patient as the primary consideration. Hospitals deal with life and
the quality of life for individuals and cannot become a battleground
for opposing forces.

This book, for the first time, objectively and factually, without
emotion and without taking of sides, details for both administrator
and employee their responsibilities and obligations under the National
Labor Relations Act. It sets forth, for the administrator and the hospital
management team, a clear picture of their roles and the need to take
a fresh look at their employee relations program regardless of unionization. For technicians, professional people, and other hospital workers,
the book clearly delineates their responsibilities and the advantages and
disadvantages of union organization.

It is an invaluable tool for both groups in confronting the benefits
and drawbacks they face today in this new era of employee relations.

Stephen M. Morris

The basic premise that employees' rights to organize must be acknowledged is inherent in a belief in a democratic society. There is no question that philosophical differences over the Economic and General Welfare program have always been in existence in the American Nurses' Association and are still present, even though the program has been in existence since the late 1940's. However, the House of Delegates at each biennium convention of the association has reaffirmed its support of this very important program. While the direction of the program and the structure to accommodate it may have changed, the support is still there.

It was a privilege for me to be able to review this text before publication. The authors have written a factual, objective book on labor relations in the health care field. The reasons that collective action and unionization are emotionally charged concepts, and why they should not be, are explained very well. Likewise, the "Points for Reflection" at the end of each chapter are appropriate and important ones. I commend the authors for this book and trust that those who read it will benefit.

Rosamond C. Gabrielson

The effective delivery of health care is important to every member of society. When the delivery system faces challenges to its performance, every practitioner, educator, and student must know the nature and causes of the potential disruptions.

In the long history of health care few developments have held a potential for disruption as significant as collective action by employees. Just the word *union* too often causes administrators and employees to envision strikes — strikes that may very well interrupt necessary medical treatment. To virtually all providers of health care, such disruptions are abhorrent. Patients suffer; the health care facility loses revenue; and employees are subjected to the economic and emotional vicissitudes of a work stoppage.

Although federal legislation has built in safeguards to minimize these interruptions, each participant in labor-management relations has power. And power — the ability to limit another's alternatives — is most dangerous in the hands of the uninformed. The best hope for society, clients (patients), and health care providers is that the holders of this power have a clear, unbiased understanding of labor relations. In the final analysis it is not the laws but the people themselves who determine how the power of collective action is used or abused.

To aid practitioners and other students of health care, this book sets forth the laws, procedures, and techniques that have proved successful for administrators and for employees' representatives in the conduct of collective action. The reasons and emotions behind these practices are also explored to give a more complete understanding of the entire labor relations process. The causes of union membership and nonmembership are explained; and the unique quandary faced by professionals, the results of emotional reactions, and the rights of union members are also considered.

These topics and others are presented from a position of "active" neutrality. Neither of us thinks that administrators or employee leaders are inherently right. Therefore, inappropriate and illegal behaviors are so labeled, irrespective of who is culpable. This active neutrality not only reflects our own views but is used to contrast the inherent power relationships that emerge in any labor-management association. If a meaningful comprehension of labor relations is to exist, it is imperative that each health care provider understands that the foundation of every labor-management relationship is the relative power of the participants.

W. B. W.
C. A. L.

Tempe, Arizona

Acknowledgments

It is impossible to acknowledge all the individuals who have influenced the writing of this book. Family, professors, friends, and practitioners — all have greatly contributed to our thinking and our individual and professional growth.

We thank Colene Schested, Assistant Professor, Arizona State University, for initiating the project that brought the authors together. Dr. Sarah Archer, Assistant Professor, University of California at San Francisco; Rosemarie Sandling, Assistant Professor, Arizona State University; Mr. Edward Sandling; and Mr. Christopher Campbell, Editor, Little, Brown and Company: each gave moral support and guidance at the right moments.

Technical assistance, questions, issues, and challenges were offered to us by Dr. Dan L. Dearen, Vice President, Human Resources and Development; Mr. James R. Baken, Director of Employee Relations; and Mr. Michael Quinn, Executive Director of Personnel Management Services,. each of Samaritan Health Service, Phoenix, Arizona. Mrs. Hazel Bennett, Executive Director, Arizona Nurses Association, not only offered assistance and challenges but, fortunately for us, she gathered information about both sides of the issues and made sure we listened. Mr. Murray A. Gordon, Esq., Legal Counsel to the American Nurses' Association, provided us with valuable material on many issues. To Ms. Rosamond C. Gabrielson and Mr. Stephen M. Morris goes our gratitude for taking the time to review and comment on the manuscript. To have two such leaders in the health care field prepare forewords to our text is an honor that we gratefully acknowledge.

We thank Dr. Robert Wright of Robert Wright and Associates and Professor Keith Davis of Arizona State University who provided needed insights into the complexities of developing a book. We also thank Mary Tallman who typed the manuscript, and, of course, thanks to Mrs. June Besson, who knows only too well the contribution she has made. To Linda Werther, for her support, patience, and objectivity, we give love and appreciation.

To each of these people we express our sincere gratitude and our recognition of their valuable contributions.

W. B. W.
C. A. L.

Tempe, Arizona

Contents

Labor Relations in the Health Professions

The Distribution of Power

The greater the power, the more dangerous the abuse.
— *Edmund Burke*

Labor relations affects every provider of health care because it encompasses the entire range of employment laws, administrative motivations, employee needs, professional standards, collective actions, legal rights, and individual responsibilities.

Each of these considerations exists within every facility of the health care industry. These factors compound the inherently complicated process of providing care. Furthermore, this complexity is amplified in importance by the extreme interdependence of providers and clients within the health care delivery system. The result is the most complex employee-employer relationship within the most complex industry of the twentieth century.

SOURCES OF POWER

The intricacy of health care delivery would degenerate into chaos if it were not for a precarious balance of power. It is the power of providers (administrators, professionals, technocrats, and unskilled workers), government regulations, and clients that holds the system together. Without a distribution of power among the participants, the system would not — in fact, could not — function.

Each provider possesses power in every employment relationship. The power of administrators, for example, acts as a constraint on the power of nurses and vice versa. Without these countervailing forces, order is replaced with confusion and the technical, financial, and physical resources of the system are misused and depleted.

Administrators have power through authority. This authority comes from the administrator's position within a specific institution. The authority of each manager and submanager is delegated by superiors in accordance with the responsibilities of each position [7]. This authority, however, is tenuous. It is based upon the assumption that the manager's subordinates will acquiesce to valid commands. Even other sources of power — such as a manager's expertise or governmentally bestowed rights — are dependent upon this acquiescence.

The power of nonadministrative personnel is derived from three sources. One is the acceptance or rejection of managerial orders. Although the consequences of a direct refusal to submit to administrative authority make this an alternative of last resort, it is one method by which nonadministrative providers can assert power. More often, however, a refusal to comply with orders is in the form of indirect actions or inactions that limit managerial power without confronting it. A second source of power is ability. Knowledge gives an individual power, especially in the highly specialized and interdependent health care network. Administrators often find their role in health care to be that of a coordinator more than that of a direct manager simply because they do not know a task as well as a subordinate does. The use of direct authority in these situations becomes unnecessary and counterproductive. The final source of employee power results from governmentally imposed constraints upon the employer [8].

External Sources

Health care is a pervasive system with strong societal implications. Virtually every citizen is dependent upon this industry to such an extent that governmental involvement is appropriate. To assure that a certain level of service is provided, legislatures, courts, and governmental agencies regulate the delivery of health care through a myriad of constraints. Some of the regulations concern patient care and staff qualifications. Of primary importance to the examination of labor relations, however, are the rules that shape the relationship between the employees and the organization — or, more simply, the employment relationship. These will be explained in more detail in subsequent chapters. Labor laws and their interpretation present administrators with a long list of prohibitions, the purpose of which is to grant workers certain rights. These rights and their associated responsibilities enable nonadministrative personnel to form or not to form unions free of management interference. Other laws make discrimination based upon sex, age, race, religion, and national origin illegal. Still other laws force the employer to provide a safe working environment. Each of these governmental constraints gives nonmanagerial employees the power to invoke government intervention.

Clients also have power. Theirs is the power of consumers to direct their expenditures according to the services they seek. Although clients have seldom used their economic power over health care institutions, they have, nevertheless, the potential to demand that services be made accessible, acceptable, and accountable. This source of power will grow when and if clients exercise their right to be involved and informed about how care is offered [6].

Clients also have the political power to pressure legislatures into adding constraints on health care practitioners. Likewise, suits can be used to bring the weight of the courts to bear on the system. Unlike consumer power, judicial and political power have been effectively used. And, even when no court actions or legislative enactments occur, the potential for such developments constrains providers and makes clients powerful [4]. The sometimes excessive use of diagnostic tests to forestall malpractice suits provides a current example.

Each of the participants in the health system — managers, employees, government, and clients — exercises some control over health care employment relationships, because each has power. This power is not without bounds. It is limited for each participant by the power of others in the relationship. Labor relations is, therefore, a study of controlled power.

HISTORICAL EVOLUTION OF POWER RELATIONSHIPS

The present power context did not suddenly emerge. Its current state of development has evolved largely during the last fifty years.

For several millennia the need to marshal human, technological, financial, and physical resources in order to deliver health care was the sole responsibility of the physician. As the vertical family unit lessened in importance, care for the sick increasingly became a societal burden. Out of humanitarian and charitable reasons, hospitals began to be built. Initially they were little more than repositories for the dying. As technology and medical knowledge grew, the hospital and other health care institutions slowly were transformed from repositories for the dying into reservoirs of specialized skills and machines. Institutions came to play a growing role in the delivery of health care. The personnel in these facilities underwent a parallel change. Volunteers gave way to trained professionals. As time progressed, existing professionals became more specialized and new ones evolved. Increased specialization and a growing number of support personnel created an exceedingly complex health care delivery system. As a result, administrators were needed to coordinate these human, financial, and technological resources yet, even as administrators gained power, other forces were emerging to diffuse the administrators' authority.

PRESENT EMPLOYEE SOPHISTICATION

Doctors and nurses who once met nearly all patient needs are now supplemented with a growing cadre of professional and auxiliary personnel. Although these developments improve the possible range of health care, they further obscure traditional lines of authority. Doctors and nurses must now integrate information from a multiplicity of sources. Technologists, staff specialists, hospital policies, and intricate medical procedures all must be considered.

These changes require a new type of health care worker — one with advanced training. Although this is obvious today, it is a radical departure from half a century ago. When health care facilities existed primarily to comfort (not cure) the sick, the major requirement for employment was concern. Today concern is an important component, but the determinant of employment, for all but the most menial jobs, is ability. Ability or skill level is partially related to education. This means that one passport to employment in the health care field is a formal education.

Prior to this trend those who worked in health care were fairly easily dichotomized into professional providers, who had wide discretion in patient care, and the unskilled. Today there is a third category — technocrats. Technocrats are highly trained experts who are each responsible for a specific area of health care. They are, in their own right, professionals. They do not, however, have the broad responsibility for client care that doctors and nurses do.

Advanced educational requirements, years of study, and the proliferation of technocrats and other professionals have changed the character of health care providers. Although still influenced by humanitarian considerations, they are primarily employees. Their motivations include more than just the esteem needs of achievement and recognition derived from helping others. They are also motivated to work by economic and interpersonal needs. Unlike their predecessors these employees demand more than just humanitarian satisfactions.

Meeting these diverse motivations is made even more difficult for management by the heterogeneous composition of the employees. Except for the housekeeping and orderly functions, most providers fifty years ago were middle-class workers. The menial tasks were relegated to employees from lower social strata. Those who provided direct health care were likely to be from a social background that permitted advanced education or free voluntary assistance. Economic considerations were less important. With education as the passport to today's jobs in the health care field, the composition of the work force is a blend of all social strata. Moreover these different backgrounds pervade all positions held by providers — unskilled, technical, and professional.

When the multiple economic, social, and esteem needs of today's health care workers are not satisfied, the repercussions reverberate throughout the facility. Whether employees resign, become less productive, or form unions, all these responses create problems that diminish the quality of health care. Sooner or later these problems require action by management. If that action does not result in sufficient and properly distributed rewards, the employees take action. That is, they assert their power.

SOCIAL CLIMATE FOR COLLECTIVE ACTION

As recently as fifty years ago there were essentially no government regulations affecting the employment relationship in health care facilities. Administrators were virtually masters of all they surveyed. Today this is being challenged. Employees are becoming knowledgeable in labor-management relations and demanding a share in the administrator's

authority. Well-intentioned but incapable administrators who resist
sharing power are further provoking the challenge. The size and complexity of many health care institutions contribute to discontent. The
acceptance of collective action by employees and the public also helps
to challenge old patterns of authority.

Since the health care industry was perceived by many government
officials to be largely a collection of charitable organizations, employment-related laws typically contained exemptions for health care institutions, especially for nonprofit facilities. This was particularly true of laws
designed to further union organization. Nevertheless the power of employees within the health care system grew simply because of the growing
complexities and specialization of health care.

Even in the absence of laws to protect employees, this power occasionally erupted into open conflict that impaired the delivery of health
services within the community. Nonadministrative providers banded
together and demanded that power be shared as the quid pro quo for
returning to work. The operation of a health care facility under such
circumstances became largely a custodial affair; the interdependency
and overwhelming complexity of health services made it virtually impossible to deliver care when providers withdrew. Government action to
control disruptions became inevitable.

Government Intervention

In 1935 several laws were enacted to pull the country out of the Great
Depression. One of these laws was the National Labor Relations Act
(NLRA). It emerged from the economic hypothesis that unions would
prevent employers from cutting the wages of workers; that this would
result in higher worker incomes; that spending would then increase; and
that this additional spending would allow the country to pull out of the
depression. Unfortunately, economic history has shown this reasoning
to be false because many employers who could not reduce wages went
bankrupt.

Nevertheless, the power of employers had to be limited to achieve
the federal government's objective of increased unionization. No longer
could employers legally fire employees who sought to unionize. The
National Labor Relations Board (NLRB), created by the NLRA, was
empowered to investigate and initiate administrative proceedings against

those employers who violated the law. If NLRB administrative actions did not succeed in curtailing the illegal acts, court action was pursued.

The NLRA was clearly biased, as it listed only employer violations. Twelve years later, in 1947, the National Labor Relations Act was substantially amended and became known as the Taft-Hartley Act. The Taft-Hartley Act, or, as it is legally entitled, the Labor Management Relations Act, listed prohibitions for·unions.

This law came about for several reasons. First, some unions (primarily in the coal industry) struck during the war. In the mind of the public these actions were generalized to the entire union movement, and organized labor suffered the first of its two major public relations blunders. Second, immediately following World War II the nation experienced the most rapid inflation in its history, and unions were blamed. Their failure to explain the true causes* of this inflation constituted their second major public relations failure. The third reason for the Taft-Hartley Act was that the previous act was wholly one-sided. (The initial union bias in the law may have been reasonable at that time, since in 1935 unions were largely feeble organizations except in the fields of construction and mining.)

Twelve years later, 1959, a third modification was made to these laws: The Labor-Management Reporting and Disclosure Act. This act, also known as the Landrum-Griffin Act, had two purposes. First, it was designed to curb union abuses that had been documented by the McClelland Committee in the previous Congress. The result was the so-called Union Members' Bill of Rights. Safeguards against corrupt financial and election procedures employed by a few unions was the goal of this bill of rights. The other purpose of the law was to make adjustments in the Taft-Hartley Act.

---

*The inflation following World War II was the result of the war and government policy. The war diverted the factories from consumer to war goods manufacturing. Cars, appliances, and other consumer goods were simply not available. Unemployment was virtually eliminated by massive government deficits to pay for war goods. These debts were financed by war bonds that could easily be converted into cash. The result was a population flush with cash (or near-cash instruments). When price and wage controls were removed by President Truman, the accumulated savings of four years were sent chasing too few goods. (This is a classic example of demand-pull inflation.) Unions, free to strike legally, tried to keep up with inflation, and countless strikes resulted when employers balked. Since massive strikes and high inflation rates were occurring simultaneously, the inference drawn by politicians and the public was that unions caused the inflation. In fact, they did not; the culprit was government policy.

The 1947 act contained an exemption for nonprofit health care institutions. Due to the unique role of the nonprofit health institutions and considerable lobbying by employer representatives, this exemption persisted. Public Law 93-360, the Nonprofit Health Care Amendments to the Taft-Hartley Act, became effective on August 25, 1974, and put an end to this exemption. The 1974 law did two things. First, it made nonprofit health care facilities subject to the national labor laws. It assured covered employees the right to join or refrain from joining with others to form a union. Second, the law created special notification procedures that must precede any strike action. (The details of the Labor Management Relations Act, as amended, will be explained in Chapter 4. The notification process will be presented in Chapter 9.)

The desperation spawned by the depression, the growing acceptance of collective action by society, and past labor and management abuses caused labor relations laws to come into being. These laws are important because they are the legal framework that shapes the employment relationship. As is the case with most legislation, these laws really did not usher in a new era. Health care providers (and others) were already taking collective action. The passage of this legislation was merely a government acknowledgment of ongoing activities. Admittedly, however, these laws (collectively known as the Labor Management Relations Act, as amended) did lead to increased unionization in many industries.

The Present Framework

Technological advances are constantly occurring, resulting in increased specialization. A stream of NLRB, court, and legislative decrees is produced each year. Societal attitudes and managerial techniques continue to change. What each of these observations means is that health care labor relations is dynamic. The different bases of power change; they are in a constant state of flux.

At present the balance of power is such that nonadministrative employees have a federally guaranteed right to form unions. Although management is not compelled to accept this development in silence, the employer may not undertake any direct or indirect actions that deny employee wishes to unionize.

With this right of employees to organize, however, there are responsibilities [8]. Some forms of collective action against the employer may violate labor laws. Unionzation does not reduce obligations to clients nor accountability to management. Even more significantly for some, it requires an assessment of individual loyalties. Professional employees who serve in management capacities have already found their employers reluctant to support membership in professional organizations. In fact some manager-professionals have been required to withdraw from professional associations when their associations have undertaken collective action against an employer.

Employees who become members of collective action groups typically find that they obtain new power. This power is offset in part, however, by the addition of new constraints: the labor-management agreement. The agreement or contract specifies — often in considerable detail — prohibited and required actions. The employment realtionship becomes more formalized. The document serves as a limit on management *and* workers. In fact wherever power exists within labor relations, there is almost certainly a countervailing power, often in the form of a new responsibility. Failure to use a new power diligently, even in the absence of a balancing power or responsibility, leads to a reaction. The reaction is a constraint on the power. The limitation is imposed by some other participant in the labor-management relationship.

When administrators consistently abuse their power throughout an entire industry, the reaction is government controls [8]. These may come in the form of court orders, legislative enactments, or, more commonly, the rulings of a government agency [8]. If administrative power is consistently misused in the context of a single employment relationship, collective action by the employees is the primary method of restoring the power balance.

Power, therefore, does not exist in a vacuum. Instead its use creates a dependency relationship. Each participant is dependent upon the other. Employees depend upon administrators for jobs and wages; administrators rely upon subordinates to provide necessary services; clients rely on both for health care; and the government needs providers to maintain the health of the citizenry.

Any party that ignores this power-dependency relationship does so at its own peril [2]. If administrators bring too much power to bear against workers, the workers may organize. If organized, they may strike. Strikes, especially long ones, lead to the loss of personnel. Moreover those employees that quit are often the most capable ones, who readily find jobs because of their exceptional abilities. Besides the cost of replacement (e.g., recruiting, training, and record keeping), organizational performance suffers, since replacements are not as efficient until they become oriented. Furthermore disruptions in service lead to underutilization of facilities. Empty beds generate no revenue, only costs.

In the same manner the overuse of power by employee organizations has negative repercussions. A health care facility with a depleted budget cannot provide its personnel with better benefits, higher wages, or improved working conditions. Needless work rules, overworked complaint mechanisms, and trivial demands that are backed by employee power make the administrative system insensitive to necessary changes. At the same time these demands further diminish finite resources that would otherwise be available for wages and benefits.

Even government ignores the power-dependency relationship at its own expense. The proliferation of laws, agency decisions, and court rulings adds a complex maze of controls to the delivery of health care. Any practitioner who has ever completed Medicare reports, developed an affirmative action plan, or complied with other government requirements realizes the time and costs involved. The result is higher fees for health care, which are translated into politically unacceptable higher inflation rates and government expenditures.

For health care providers there is an even more important consideration. If the balance between power and dependency becomes too one-sided, Congress will modify the rules under which the parties must operate. The history of labor relations legislation is replete with amendments designed to redress power imbalances. By including nonprofit health care facilities under the nation's labor laws, Congress has gone on record indicating its willingness to experiment to assure health care delivery to the public. Should employee groups or administrators consistently exercise too much power, they will find their power limited [2].

Possible future legislative restraints are examined in the last chapter of this book. The intervening chapters assess the implications of collective action by employees and the response of administrators. The role of government in labor relations and its impact on the employment relationship is explored. The methods used by employees to equalize power through collective action and the aftermath are also explained. This includes a look at labor-management negotiations and the administration of the resulting labor agreement. Strikes and the federally mandated notification procedures are a possibility whenever collective action is resorted to by workers. A separate chapter is devoted to this area. Cooperation between organized workers and management is examined because of its importance to the present and future employment relationship.

SUMMARY

Labor relations concerns every provider, because it is the study of the employment relationship. This study is made difficult in the health care field by the complexity of the industry and the relationships between the participants.

Each participant — employees, administrators, clients, and government — has power. The power of each acts as a countervailing force upon the use of power by the others. The entire labor-management context is an example of controlled power set within a web of interdependencies. The actions of every party influence the actions of the others. Nevertheless, if it were not for the distribution of power within the health care field, chaos would replace client services.

The evolution of the power distribution has been a history of declining administrative authority. The specialized knowledge of non-administrative providers has grown during recent decades. This has increased their power. Government regulations have also increased their power.

Government laws, rulings, and court decisions have resulted in a series of constraints under which administrators must discharge their responsibility of coordinating the delivery of health care. Principle among these has been the Labor Management Relations Act, as amended. It protects employees in their desire to join (or refrain from joining) unions.

The major lesson to be learned from an understanding of the power relationships is that they operate within an environment of dependency. The use and abuse of power carries with it strong implications. When power is abused, there is invariably a reaction. The response may be legal prohibitions or constraints imposed by other participants in the power relationship.

'TS FOR REFLECTION

1. Describe the power possessed by each of the participants in the employment relationship.
2. How is the power of each participant balanced by the power of the others?
3. What constraints are placed upon participant powers?
4. Discuss the implications of unlimited power in the hands of any one participant in the employment relationship.

SELECTED READINGS

1. Archer, Sarah E. Politics and Economics: How Things Really Work. In Sarah E. Archer and Ruth P. Fleshman (Eds.), *Community Health Nursing: Patterns and Practice*. North Scituate, Mass.: Duxbury Press, 1975.
2. Davis, Keith, and Robert L. Blomstrom. *Business Society and Environment: Social Power and Social Response* (3rd ed.). New York: McGraw-Hill Book Company, 1975.
3. Deloughery, Grace L., and Kristine M. Gebbie. *Political Dynamics: Impact on Nurses and Nursing*. St. Louis: C. V. Mosby Company, 1975.
4. Kahn, Si. *How People Get Power*. New York: McGraw-Hill Book Company, 1970.
5. Leavitt, Harold J. *Managerial Psychology* (3rd ed.). Chicago: The University of Chicago Press, 1972.
6. Lockhart, Carol A. Community Nursing Services in the Home. In Sarah E. Archer and Ruth P. Fleshman (Eds.), *Community Health Nursing: Patterns and Practice*. North Scituate, Mass.: Duxbury Press, 1975.
7. Simon, Herbert A. Authority. In John H. Turner, Alan C. Filley, and Robert J. House (Eds.), *Studies In Managerial Process and Organizational Behavior*. Glenview, Ill.: Scott, Foresman and Company, 1972.
8. Werther, William B., Jr. Government control v. corporate ingenuity. *Labor Law Journal* 26:360, 1975.

2

Unions: Structure and Member Rights

Knowledge itself is power.
  — Francis Bacon

Collective action is an emotionally charged topic. Most people respond to discussions of collective action with a reaction born of hearsay, conventional wisdom, and ignorance, but with little objectivity. They perceive selectively, accepting only information that reinforces previous conceptions (or misconceptions). Such reactions are particularly surprising in an industry with a high concentration of professionals. If providers applied the same unemotional objectivity that they rely on in their work to the study of collective action, animosity and morale problems would subside. Admittedly participants would still have different perspectives and arrive at different conclusions. In the absence of emotionalism, however, administrators and employees could more effectively obtain their goals and their common objective of improved health care delivery.

The implications of collective action are of concern to administrators and employees alike. An objective assessment of collective action requires an understanding of its basic components. This chapter will delineate the structure of unions and professional associations and the roles, rights, and responsibilities emerging from concerted efforts. Chapter 3 will then explore the advantages and disadvantages of collective action.

EMPLOYEE ORGANIZATIONS

The term *union* has strong emotional connotations. This has led to countless euphemistic substitutes. Some of the more common synonyms are *employee organizations, collective action groups, labor organizations, employee associations,* and even *professional associations.* These terms are used interchangeably. Although the term *professional association* denotes groups that function solely to further the competency of members or the stature of the profession, those that bargain or police agreements between their members and employers are acting as unions. Professional associations are attempting to cope with this dilemma by establishing separate divisions for professional advancement and collective action. This tactic seeks to allow members of management to retain their affiliation with the professional division. The American Nurses' Association's Commission on Economic and General Welfare is an example of a collective action division within a professional association. Nevertheless, as unpalatable as the term *union* may be, groups that negotiate or enforce labor agreements are unions.

There are minor differences between unions, whatever their names, but several common characteristics stand out. All unions exist to improve wages, hours, and working conditions [2]. (These issues will be presented in Chapter 7.) Health care unions are constrained by a common body of law. (These legal regulations are explained in Chapter 4.) Among unions in the United States, there are similarities in organizational structure and the rights of members. These characteristics are fundamental to assessing collective action and will be discussed in the remainder of this chapter.

UNION ORGANIZATIONAL STRUCTURE

Labor organizations do vary in their organizational design, but the differences are not substantive. Variations center around classification and labeling of offices. Professional associations have more significant differences and will be discussed separately.

Union efforts occur at three levels: the local organization, the national organization, and the federation. Each level affects providers directly and indirectly. The most observable influence results from the local organization.

Locals

Local organizations – or, as they are more commonly called, *locals* – are the backbone of the union movement. It is from membership in individual locals that all union power originates.

For most nonmembers the union means a large organization run from New York or Washington, D. C., dictating what members will and will not do. For some, it is "outsiders" establishing another list of rules; it simply becomes a new master to serve. These beliefs overlook the grassroots nature of collective action.

In any organization with a union, including a health care facility, the work-place rules are established between management and the employees' representatives. Through collective bargaining negotiations at the local level (by local people) the wages, hours, work rules, and other conditions of employment are set down. Outside influence is minimal; suggestions from representatives of national bodies are usually advisory and welcomed by leaders and members alike. In fact, negotiations are only conducted by national bodies when the employer operates facilities on a nationwide basis. Even then, local negotiations still occur.

The local organization functions with several key offices and committees. Diagrammatically these can be seen in Figure 1. The president is the principal official of the local. Financial affairs and record keeping

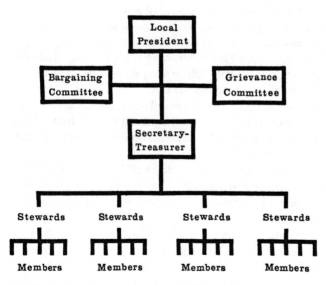

Figure 1   Local union organizational structure.

are delegated to the combined office of secretary-treasurer except in large locals, in which these activities may be split. Stewards are the employees' day-to-day contact with the union. It is through the stewards that formal complaints or grievances are made against management. The stewards police the labor contract and ensure that managers do not violate its provisions [1].

When a steward cannot get a company supervisor to comply with the contract, the grievance is taken to the next higher level of management. If there is still no satisfaction, the complaint is turned over to a grievance committee. The committee usually consists of the union president as chairperson, the secretary-treasurer, and some or all of the stewards. The local's constitution and bylaws determine the exact composition of the grievance team.

The bargaining committee may have the same mix of officers and members as the grievance committee. This, too, is controlled by the constitution and bylaws. Two noteworthy additional members are a lawyer and a national representative. The negotiation of the contract is a complex matter that results in a legal document. Since union officials are unlikely to be qualified labor attorneys, it is usual to retain a labor lawyer.

If the local bargaining team is experienced and knowledgeable, the representative of the national union (if the local is affiliated to one) merely acts as an observer. Under most circumstances the bargaining team is neither sophisticated nor experienced in negotiations. Here the representative can provide expert advice and judgment based on experience and research conducted by the parent body. In fact, since the representative is often the most experienced negotiator, local officials may allow the rep actually to conduct the negotiations for them. Even when this happens, the goals of the negotiations are determined by the local leaders and members [1].

Nothing in the law requires the local to be affiliated with a national union. Many independent locals exist. They hire or develop their own experts and receive no assistance from national unions. Independent locals are maintained to alleviate fears that "outsiders" will influence proceedings or to avoid the payment of dues beyond those needed to run the local. Since local and national dues typically are equivalent to one or two hours' pay a month, the money saved by not affiliating with a national union is modest compared to the cost of services that independent locals must secure in the open market.

National Unions

The power of the national unions is based solely upon the support of their affiliated locals. It is through the local unions that the national receives dues — the revenue needed to run the organization. Furthermore the larger the number of people affiliated with it, the more lobbying and political clout the national union has with government officials. National bodies have existed for over a century because of common concerns among employees. Many problems — safety, minimum wages, industry regulations — are faced by members who work for different employers. No one local can deal effectively with such sweeping issues. However, if they are joined together into nationwide organizations, the national can use resources from all locals to find and gain solutions. If affiliated locals also exist in Canada, the national union usually is called an *international* union but functions the same way.

As national unions have grown, they have been able to provide a varied list of services to locals. Lobbying at the national level — at least from the union perspective — is one way to solve problems transcending the individual employer-local relationships. The Occupational Safety and Health Act was vigorously lobbied for by many national unions, for example. Other services offered to affiliated locals include research results, expert opinions, economic forecasts, model constitutions and bylaws, and training.

The most valuable assistance is rendered through the field representative. Besides assisting with negotiations, the rep contributes to the organization of new locals, guides local leaders through the complexities of securing a government-controlled election, and may even protect members from illegal acts by obtaining government investigations of wrongdoing.

To carry on these functions, national unions are organized along the lines depicted in Figure 2. At a convention, representatives from the locals elect the executive officers and members to the executive board. The executive board advises the executive officers. The board's composition normally includes the executive and regional officers of the union. Frequently these boards merely reflect the wishes of the president. It is the president, through popularity with convention delegates and control of in-house newpapers and publications — who largely determines nominations to the executive board. The president is the spokesman for the national and responsible for administrative appointments throughout its

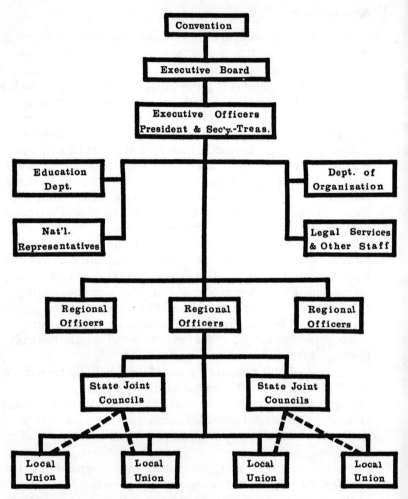

Figure 2   National union organizational structure.

structure. The secretary-treasurer's role can be either a ceremonial position of little importance or an important administrative post that supervises the day-to-day operations of the national.

The national's staff departments are the primary sources of assistance to the locals. The national representatives form one department at the headquarters (as shown) or report directly to the regional officers. They serve as liaison between the national and local organizations. The education department traditionally provides training to members in the locals. This may be through formal seminars at national headquarters or in regional offices around the country. Sometimes the education department is simply a source of written documents designed to keep local officials informed on economic, political, and other items of interest. The department of organization, if separate from the national representatives, exists to "organize the unorganized." It will send (unsolicited or on request) trained union organizers to help workers form a union. The department of legal services offers expert advice and research to assist locals in dealing with difficult legal issues. Other staff services may include auxiliary groups for retired members, legislative lobbies, public relations, accounting and finance, and related functions typical of any large organization.

Federations

At present the only significant federation is the *American Federation of Labor and Congress of Industrial Organizations* (AFL-CIO). Its power is based upon the national unions affiliated with it. Each of these national unions contributes a share of its dues through a per capita tax to the AFL-CIO. The AFL-CIO exists to assist the entire labor movement with coordination and resolution of problems confronting all organized workers. Other coalitions, past and present, have been formed when several national unions have perceived joint action to be in their mutual benefit. The Coalition of Postal Employees and the Alliance for Labor Action are two examples.

Problems affecting national unions are job safety, retirement, and discrimination, to mention a few. On each of these issues the AFL-CIO has vigorously lobbied and brought the power of its millions of members to bear. These actions have facilitated the passage of numerous employment-related laws.

The AFL-CIO provides coordination for the union movement through its organizational structure. As shown in Figure 3 the biennial convention is the nominal means of determining the leaders [9]. Although the convention officially elects the executive officers and the executive council, the president largely controls the nomination process. Members

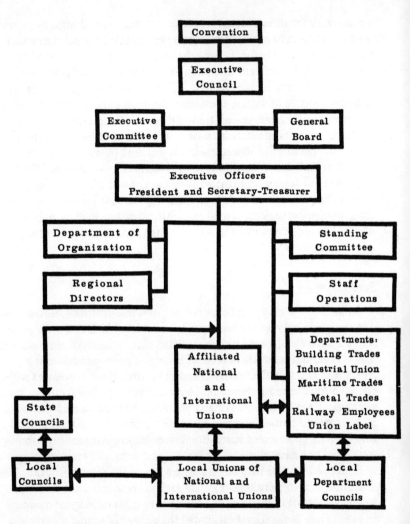

Figure 3   Organizational structure of the AFL-CIO.

of the executive council are also members of the general board; the chief of every affiliated union and constitutionally established department within the AFL-CIO is also a member of the general board. The board decides on matters referred to it from the executive council, one of which is the presidential candidate the AFL-CIO will endorse. An executive committee is selected by the executive council to meet every two months. It advises the executive officers on policy and financial matters.

The AFL-CIO headquarters has staff functions similar to those found in national unions. The division of regional directors functions to coordinate AFL-CIO activities, problems, and public relations and generally keeps the headquarters informed on developments in the field. Standing committees exist to examine issues crucial to the workers. Topics include social security, legislation, civil rights, community services, and others. The department of organization assists unionization activities in a manner similar to the way this department functions in the nationals. Staff operations attend to the internal administrative functioning of the AFL-CIO. Six departments are established by the AFL-CIO constitution to perform research and attempt to resolve intraunion and interunion difficulties. Disputes among members in different unions but within the same areas (carpenters and plumbers in building trades, for example) can be referred to the appropriate department for advice and even resolution. (Since similar conflicts in the health care field are possible, it is conceivable that a health services department may be appended to the AFL-CIO constitution.) When problems arise between allied unions and employers, these departments may help. However, assistance is normally provided by the local counterparts of the departments, the local councils.

Since each government subdivision passes its own laws and ordinances, and these may affect several different national unions, there is often a need to coordinate activity at the city, county, or state levels. This includes informing members of legal actions designed to change their rights and lobbying to modify laws in a manner favorable to the labor organizations. These functions are conducted by the affiliated state and local bodies [7].

Locals may be directly affiliated with the AFL-CIO. That is, they are not associated with any national union. This happens when the members cannot or do not wish to be affiliated with a national union but seek the services of the AFL-CIO. This sometimes occurs when the local is expelled or withdraws from a national union that is not part of the AFL-CIO.

Much of the power possessed by labor organizations comes from the strength and design of their structure. Each major external force has a corresponding internal organization to cope with it: the local negotiates with the employer; the national faces employers nationwide and problems common to all members; state and local assemblies counterbalance state and local governments; and the AFL-CIO, as well as the national unions, represents the interests of union members at the federal level.

Professional Associations

The evolution and structure of professional associations parallel those of the traditional union movement. Like unions professional associations are typically divided into three levels: district, state, and national. The primary distinction is the more significant role played by the state association.

The local districts or councils are a focus for meetings designed to further professionalism. If the district begins to represent its members in dealings with administrators, its function and structure come to resemble those of local unions. The district president becomes increasingly concerned with contract administration and negotiations. Committees to handle grievances and negotiations are formed; members are elected or appointed to positions that are equivalent to a steward in a local union. The separation of the district's interests into a professional division that focuses exclusively on improving the competency or reputation of the profession and another division that conducts labor-management relations attempts to mesh the needs of administrative and staff professionals.

In the health care field, the state association rather than the national acts as the primary source of assistance for the local districts. It provides legal counsel, representatives to assist with organizing and negotiations, research, model constitutions and bylaws, lobbying, and many of the other services typically provided for local unions by the national. The state association contains professional interest groups, divisions on professional practices, and standing committees devoted to issues of concern in the profession. Since most laws that affect health care professionals are state enacted, the evolution of professional associations has concentrated power in the state associations.

The national association plays a role similar to that of the AFL-CIO. Its primary functions are to lobby at the national level, provide research information, and further the interests of its affiliated state bodies. It, too, maintains standing committees, divisions on professional practices, and interest groups or occupational forums.

As is the case with unions, the membership at each level elects the officers at meetings or conventions of delegates. One notable difference is that these leaders normally retire from office after their tour of duty (unlike union officers, who often perpetuate themselves in office).

Professional health care associations and more traditional unions have essentially the same structure. When a professional association begins to represent its members through negotiations with health care administrators, it becomes a union and falls under the legal constraints on unions [4].

RIGHTS OF MEMBERS

Members of unions have rights and responsibilities as a result of their association with others [5]. One of the sources of these rights is the Labor Management Relations Act, as amended. This law controls employers and labor organizations in their relationships with each other and employees. As explained in Chapter 4, it is an important source of rights. Another basis of rights and responsibilities is derived from the labor-management contract between the union and the employer. Wage rates, fringe benefits, seniority provisions, overtime allocation procedures, employee duties, and other issues are specified in the contract. (The discussion of contract negotiations in Chapter 7 expands on these topics.) A third source of rights and responsibilities is the union constitution and bylaws. These documents vary widely. Most contain provisions to ensure fair elections of officers, equal representation for members in the processing of grievances, and equitable methods of levying dues and special assessments. Many of the safeguards written into union constitutions are required by the fourth source of member's rights: The Labor-Management Reporting and Disclosure Act (LMRDA).

The Labor-Management Reporting and Disclosure Act of 1959 was passed by Congress to guarantee that certain basic rights and freedoms would not be denied union members. It provided for

the reporting and disclosure of certain financial transactions and administrative practices of labor organizations and employers, to prevent abuses in the administration of trusteeships by labor organizations, to provide standards with respect to the election of officers of labor organizations, and for other purposes.

Title I of the LMRDA is referred to as the "Bill of Rights of Union Members." It contains provisions that are enforced by the Labor-Management Services Administration under the Secretary of Labor [3]. When these rights are not honored, the aggrieved may bring suit against the union or union leaders in federal district courts [8].

Equality

Any labor organization's constitution and bylaws may specify limitations on member behavior and election rights. If the provisions are reasonable and fairly administered these limitations are not abridged by LMRDA. Specifically the act requires that every union member have equal privileges in nominating and voting for union officials. Furthermore attendance and participation in general membership meetings must be open to all members in good standing.

Freedom of Speech

Again the law recognizes that unions may pass and enforce reasonable rules limiting member conduct that interferes with union responsibilities and contracts. For example, a union may fine members who intentionally disrupt gatherings of union members. Subject to reasonable rules that guide union meetings, however, members have the right to express their opinions and meet with others.

Assessments

Union dues, special assessments, and initiation fees can be raised only in accordance with the provisions of the LMRDA. Permanent changes in these charges can be made by a majority vote via a secret ballot election, by a referendum of all members in good standing, or by delegates to a convention of the national union. A national's executive board can, by majority vote, raise these charges temporarily until the next regular convention, if the constitution and bylaws bestow this power upon them.

Suits

When a member has a grievance against the labor organization or its leaders, the law anticipates that the individual will first exhaust internal union remedies or procedures. Once these remedies are exhausted (or after four months of pursuing them), the member may bring suit, appear as a witness, communicate with government officials, or take any other reasonable action designed to secure redress. The union may not restrict this right.

Arbitrary Actions

Except for the nonpayment of dues a member cannot be expelled from the union without due process. This means that the individual must be served with specific written charges, be provided a reasonable time to prepare a defense, and be granted a complete and fair hearing. Otherwise the aggrieved may file charges in a district court.

Contract Copies

Anyone who is represented by the union is entitled to a copy, upon request, of every labor-management contract that affects employee rights. This applies to all members of the local as well as to others who are represented by the union but are not dues-paying members.

Other Rights

Other sections of the LMRDA extend additional rights to members. The information contained in union reports filed with the government under the LMRDA must be made available to all members. If they show good cause, members may look at other union records and reports. (Copies of union reports may be examined at area offices of the Labor-Management Services Administration for a nominal fee.)

Occasionally a parent body removes officials from office. Although such moves are presumably intended to protect the interests of the union, opportunities for abuse are present. Historically, several well-known union leaders have used this technique to ensure the loyalty of local officials. To prevent abuses of this power, the LMRDA permits local officials to be removed from office only in accordance with the parent body's constitution and bylaws. Even then, only the following reasons are considered appropriate:

1. To restore democratic rights to members.
2. To eliminate corruption.
3. To guarantee the performance of the labor contract or other duties required of the employee's representative.
4. To discharge any other legitimate goals of the labor organization.

This removal process results in a trusteeship, which is presumed to be invalid under LMRDA if it lasts more than eighteen months.

The LMRDA requires the use of democratic election procedures. The law lists certain practices that must be followed:

1. Every member in good standing must be able to nominate candidates and run for election.
2. Secret-ballot elections must be used to elect local officials and delegates to representative assemblies and conventions.
3. Each member in good standing, without discrimination, must be allowed to vote and support candidates.
4. Each candidate is permitted to have an observer at all polling and counting stations.
5. Members are entitled to fifteen days' notice of an election.
6. Election results must be made known by locals.
7. Records of the election must be preserved for one year and safeguards must be used to ensure a fair election.
8. The election must be conducted in accordance with the union constitution and bylaws, as long as these provisions are consistent with the law.
9. Candidates are to have equal access to membership lists.
10. Union funds may not be used by any candidate to assist the candidacy of any individual seeking union office.
11. Officers must be elected every five years in national and international unions, delegates to representative assemblies must be elected every four years, and local officials must be elected every three years.

These election requirements of the LMRDA apply only to the election of regular officers. Interim leaders can be elected without adherence to these regulations.

The rights contained in the LMRDA are protected by a provision in the law that prohibits anyone from disciplining or discriminating against a member who exercises these rights. Moreover, anyone who resorts to violence to interfere with these rights is subject to a $1000 fine and up to one year of imprisonment.

Unions are democratic institutions set up to reflect the wishes of the members [6]. When leaders within the labor organization misuse their power in dealing with members, the LMRDA provides recourse to aggrieved members who have not found satisfaction within the union. The Labor-Management Services Administration has field offices in major metropolitan areas. This agency exists in part to guarantee the rights under LMRDA. If problems are within its jurisdiction, it will investigate and prosecute. Otherwise it can advise aggrieved employees on how to obtain redress — usually through a federal district court action [3].

SUMMARY

The implications of collective action are likely to be disturbing to anyone involved with the health care field. Emotional responses predicated upon preconceptions and misconceptions cloud objective thinking.

Few providers realize the grass-roots nature of labor relations. Unions are conceived of as monolithic structures totally insensitive to the needs of members. The local structure of labor organizations, however, is specifically designed to respond to the needs of the members and to local external forces. Wages, hours, and working conditions are typically resolved through local bargaining by local people. General problems of the industry are within the purview of national and international unions. Coordination among many of the national unions is provided by the AFL-CIO. When the AFL-CIO fails to meet the needs of national unions, or when the national unions fail to meet the needs of the locals, disaffiliation is always a possibility. This possibility, along with the Labor-Management Reporting and Disclosure Act, assures that the union structure will be sensitive to the needs of members.

DA imposes democratic practices upon unions. Leaders and e rights and responsibilities defined by the law. When these idged, redress can be sought through the Department of ough court action.

Unions are not perfect institutions; they have both good and bad features. Membership pressure and laws, however, curtail their most obnoxious characteristics. If these means fail, members are free to disband the union.

POINTS FOR REFLECTION

1. How may emotionalism affect a provider's assessment of collective action?
2. What are the major sources of power for locals? For national unions? For The American Federation of Labor and Congress of Industrial Organizations? For professional associations?
3. How does the organization of a union differ from that of a professional association?
4. What is the purpose of the Labor-Management Reporting and Disclosure Act?
5. What are the rights guaranteed to union members by the Labor-Management Reporting and Disclosure Act?

SELECTED READINGS

1. Alexander, Kenneth O. Union structure and bargaining structure. *Labor Law Journal* 24:164, 1973.
2. Bakke, E. Wight. *Mutual Survival, The Goal of Unions and Management.* New Haven, Conn.: Yale Labor and Management Center, 1946.
3. Brennan, Peter J. Goals of the labor department. *Labor Law Journal* 24:587, 1973.
4. Cleland, Virginia. Taft-Hartley amended: The professional model. *American Journal of Nursing* 75:2, 1975.
5. Goldberg, Arthur J. Rights and responsibilities of union members. *American Federationist* 66:15, 1959.
6. Leiserson, William M. *American Trade Union Democracy.* New York: Columbia University Press, 1959.

7. Metzger, Norman, and Dennis D. Pointer. *Labor-Management Relations in the Health Services Industry: Theory and Practice.* Washington, D. C.: Science and Health Publications, Inc., 1972.
8. U. S. Department of Labor. *Rights and Responsibilities Under the LMRDA.* Washington, D. C., 1974.
9. U. S. Department of Labor. *Directory of National and International Labor Unions in The United States, 1965* (Bulletin No. 1493). Washington, D.C., 1966.
10. Ryscavage, Paul M. Measuring union-nonunion earnings differences. *Monthly Labor Review* 97:3, 1974.

3

Implications of Collective Action

Life is the art of drawing sufficient conclusions from insufficient premises.
                                                    — Samuel Butler

An assessment of collective action requires more than an understanding of union structure and members' rights. The most significant implications emerge from the perspectives held by each provider who becomes involved in unionization. Although the reaction to unionization is unique for each participant, it is possible to discuss the general responses of different groups.

Administrators, for example, often feel betrayed when employees seek a union. The establishment of an employee organization is considered prima facie evidence of disloyalty. Yet to the worker, loyalty to the union does not mean disloyalty to management. It is not an either-or situation. Instead it is analogous to the role of a father and mother as viewed by a child: at times the child seeks the support of one parent in dealing with the other. It does not mean the child loves one parent and hates the other. Likewise, union membership may be indicative of dissatisfaction but not necessarily of disloyalty or even dislike of management.

Why then do some people join unions and others not? What reactions do administrators have to unions? These are a few of the questions that must be answered before assessing the implications of collective action.

EMPLOYEE MOTIVATIONS

The motivations of workers are so diverse that there is no single way to explain why people join or avoid unions. Instead there are many answers, with the right one always depending upon the situation. The more frequently mentioned reasons for and against union membership do provide a basis for assessment.

Joining Unions

When employees join a union, management is the primary motivator. Although few managers intentionally encourage membership, their actions — or inactions — cause employees to seek association with other workers. Managers who act capriciously, dispense discipline unfairly, fail to inform subordinates of important organizational changes, or otherwise threaten the security of workers are the principal cause of collective action. Since alternative employment is not always available, intolerable treatment leaves few remedies other than unionization. Employees may state they do not want a union, but that inequities demand action, and acting together is sometimes the only reasonable solution [1].

Another important reason for joining a union is a *union shop clause* in an existing labor contract. A union shop arrangement is an agreement between the union and the administration requiring every eligible employee to join the union within thirty or sixty days from the date of employment or the negotiation of the clause. Otherwise, the employment of the nonpaying member is usually terminated. These contractual clauses are permitted in thirty-one states.* Union shop provisions are put into labor agreements to ensure that every person who benefits from the union's efforts supports it. The motivation for joining unions under these circumstances is obvious: join or be fired.

Even when union shop clauses do not exist, present members may feel strongly about the union. When a new person starts working for the health care employer, peer pressure may force the employee to join. People who start a new job want to feel as though they belong. In this situation, peer pressure is especially effective.

Another reason for joining unions is higher wages. When the pay scale or fringe benefits of an institution is below that of similar organiza-

---

*The 19 states that do not permit a union shop clause in labor contracts are Alabama, Arizona, Arkansas, Florida, Georgia, Iowa, Kansas, Mississippi, Nebraska, Nevada, North Carolina, North Dakota, South Carolina, South Dakota, Tennessee, Texas, Utah, Virginia, and Wyoming. These are commonly referred to as *right-to-work states.*

tions (or similar jobs in the community), collective action can sometimes right the inequity [5].

Paternalistic management attempts to anticipate what the employees need (or should need) and then voluntarily satisfies that desire. This style of management may still lead to collective action. Here the motivation is not more wages. Instead collective action is caused by employees' resentment at being treated like ignorant children. Managers act as though they know what is needed and do not listen to employees. Through collective action the members hope to communicate their desires to the employer and gain some control over the rules and rewards.

Along the same lines labor organizations offer a method of airing complaints. Many health care institutions do have internally devised grievance procedures, but these do not always work fairly or effectively. Since there is no collective pressure, managers may postpone action or make a unilateral decision on grievances. Moreover, without protection from recriminations, people are often afraid to file a complaint and go over the head of the boss. A labor organization provides both the protection and the pressure [3].

These are the major motivations behind unionization. Other reasons exist: comradeship, union-provided benefits, promotion and security based on seniority instead of merit, and opportunities for leadership in the union [1]. The common denominator, however, is a need of the employee that is not being satisfied by the employer.

Avoiding Unions

Some workers have equally strong motivations for not joining unions. Again the reasons are diverse, and management plays a crucial role in the decision. Many institutions establish stringent rules that must be followed before any discipline can be administered. This assures that the system of discipline is fair. Wages and benefits are kept consistent throughout the organization and are commensurate with like positions in other facilities. At the same time management strives to maintain open communications with every worker. Such practices may result in a work environment that most employees find acceptable. Labor organizations therefore are unneeded and unwanted.

Other reasons contribute to nonmembership. Some workers have such negative opinions of unions that they would quit before becoming members. These feelings may stem from a belief that labor organizations are for blue-collar workers only. Some employees may have had unpleasant experiences with unions. Still others may have aspirations of becoming hospital administrators themselves and see union membership as detrimental to their careers.

Strikes and dues are also reasons why membership may appear undesirable. The fear of strikes is especially acute among low-paid employees, who realize that even a short strike could spell financial disaster for them. Dues may be viewed as an unnecessary expense, since the union must represent all covered employees whether members or not. Besides, if a worker is pleased with treatment from management, there will be a strong reluctance to have someone else handle representation — especially if the employees must pay for it.

Certain groups or classes of employees have always been difficult to organize. Historically women have shown less interest in unions than men [7]. Saddled with family responsibilities, women have typically lacked the career orientation and the opportunities of men. With the development of day care centers for children, the blurring of traditional work roles, and an increased consciousness of career goals, women are likely to become more active in the union movement.

Another group difficult to organize has been the employees of small companies — for example, laboratories, specialized clinics, and some nursing homes. These employees usually have closer contact with all members of management and as a result seldom seek unionization.

Although there are numerous reasons for joining or not joining an employee organization, the most significant factor is management [4]. This does not mean just top administrators and their policies. Even more crucial are first-level supervisors. How the employees' immediate boss treats them largely determines whether the workers need representation.

Administrative Reactions

Once unionization begins, management invariably asks "How can this be?" The first truly substantive answer is "supervision." First-level management often consists of senior workers or highly competent technocrats promoted from the ranks on the basis of their seniority or technical expertise. Although it may be admirable to reward longevity and technical ability, neither of these traits implies managerial competence. Thus, training supervisors in industrial and interpersonal relations is one of management's reactions to union activity.

Another typical response is the increased centralization of employee-related decisions. Discipline, promotions, raises, personnel policies, hiring, training, and similar functions are thrust upon the personnel department or the employee relations section in organizations large enough to have such staff assistance. This centralization results from the need to minimize violations of labor laws and to assure uniformity of treatment among all potential union members. Employee records must be complete in order to justify discipline. Otherwise the nearly automatic grievances that result from discipline will be won by the union [5].

Communications to the employee are normally increased. It is common to see the birth of employee newsletters, rap sessions, or suggestion systems when union activity begins. This reaction is obvious, since decisions by employees hinge upon how well management presents its case.

Administrators who act emotionally rather than rationally commit violations of the labor laws. For example, administrators may try to coerce employees by threats or rewards into not joining the union. When this occurs, it is a sign of desperation — even panic — among management. Every labor law violation gives the union organizers another example to justify the case for collective action.

Emotional reactions stem in part from managers who are used to exercising their power with little or no challenge. The union represents a threat to (or more appropriately, a throttle on) that power. What managers generally fear are restrictions on work practices. Union contracts usually specify that certain jobs will be performed only by the appropriate workers. No longer can a manager assign an employee to do something that is not part of that worker's job description. The supervisor's power is therefore limited. These restrictions, coupled with a fear that the organization will become considerably less efficient, cause management to resist unionization.

Resistance seems logical at first glance. Most people resent limitations imposed upon them. However, federal laws state that employees in profit and nonprofit health care facilities have the right to join labor organizations without management interference. This does not mean the employer must abdicate; administrators can express their opinions to workers in a noncoercive manner. It is the emotional nature of their presentations that is illogical. Administrators deal with organized groups constantly. Insurance carriers, financial institutions, medical associations, and suppliers are a few examples. When an organized group appears to represent the wishes of employees, the professional acumen that serves administrators so well in dealing with other organized groups is too often replaced with emotions. Overreactions add fuel to the organizing drive, while the administrative position is made even less tenable by legal complications.

EVALUATION OF COLLECTIVE ACTION

Employee motivations — toward membership or nonmembership — and administrative reactions offer only a partial insight into employee organizations. An assessment of the advantages and disadvantages of union membership is a prerequisite to an informed choice. Since administrators are legally bound by the wishes of their employees, the pros and cons of collective action will be evaluated from the employee perspective.

Advantages

A labor organization offers a number of advantages for health care employees. A major benefit is the equalization of power between administrators and subordinates. "Strength in numbers" and "power through solidarity" are union-organizing clichés. Nevertheless, they are accurate. The power of an employee organization is synergistic. That is, the total power is greater than the simple sum of the power possessed by each member. Individually, each employee is expendable; collectively, personnel represent the most important asset of a health care institution. When power is judiciously applied by management, there is little need to develop a countervailing force. If power is abused, then equalization is not only appropriate but advisable for employees *and* administrators. Misuse of power sooner or later results in a deterioration of morale, motivation, and ultimately performance. Such deterioration is obviously not in the best interest of the facility, its management, or its personnel. The only effective means of balancing the power relationship is to acquire the power of solidarity.

With power, other advantages are possible. Generally the benefits of power center around improved treatment. For example, a problem common to patient care personnel in continuously operating facilities is scheduling. Nonadministrative providers find that they must work four, five, six, or more weekends before their schedule entitles them to a weekend off. Holidays require a minimum staff, so days off are frequently scheduled at the convenience of supervision. Through collective bargaining, specific procedures and staffing can be established to guarantee a more systematic and equitable distribution of undesirable work shifts.

Collective action also leads to viable grievance procedures. Unlike management-designed and operated grievance mechanisms those established through the labor contract are legally enforceable. Recriminations by supervisors against subordinates who file complaints are less frequent because employees can retaliate against such discrimination by filing additional grievances. The combination of grievance procedures and bargaining is a means by which health care employees can influence the level of care provided. If administrative cost-cutting measures leave a ward understaffed or inappropriately staffed, the grievance procedure can be used to obtain a short-run solution. When an issue is critical to the ability to provide safe effective care, it can be negotiated directly into the contract between the union and the employer. Other provisions in the collective bargaining agreement can establish criteria for promotions among nonsupervisory personnel, continuing education requirements, and mandatory consultation by management prior to changes in hours or conditions of work. The more traditional benefits of higher wages, better benefits, and improved working conditions are also possible through contract negotiations [1].

An important benefit of collective action is that it permits employees to influence the rules and rule-making processes in the health care facility. When these procedures include meaningful employee involvement, internal governance is more likely to be accepted as equitable. When rules and decisions are made unilaterally by administrators, however, collective action forces management to share decision-making authority with employee representatives. This right opens the way for employees to change almost every aspect of the employment relationship and thereby affords a degree of dignity to nonadministrative providers that is too often nonexistent.

Disadvantages

Collective action is not without disadvantages. Principal among these is the recognition of an adversary relationship between administrators and subordinates. Few modern organizations require the close co-operation and teamwork found in health care facilities. The addition of new rules and regulations may impede the delivery of services. The possibility exists that the focus of efforts could shift from what is *needed* to what is *permitted*. Overly restrictive job descriptions and regulations could become ends instead of means. Although the distinction is subtle, it could lead to a deterioration in health care.

Even with the detailed notification procedures that apply to strikes in health care facilities, strikes will not be completely eliminated. The strike is a two-sided disadvantage. On one hand it impairs the per-formance of the organization. This reduces the employer's ability to meet employee demands and can seriously jeopardize patient welfare. On the other hand, strikes can severely cut down workers' income. Thus, while bringing pressure on the organization, strikes obviously hurt the strikers.

Another disadvantage of collective action is the reaction of each party to the other. When a new collective bargaining relationship is formed, both sides, labor and management, believe they need to establish their position firmly. Administrators resent their loss of power and are com-mitted to retaining their remaining rights. Collective action leaders too often attempt to correct years of neglect in the first contract. Both sides become hostile; cooperation is replaced by adamant positions. Further-more, union leaders and management representatives are usually in-experienced. The labor relations director needs to show higher level administrators that they selected the right person for the job. Union officials are normally workers who lack an understanding of just how much management can give. Furthermore the employee representatives are elected to their jobs. Like all politicians they need to satisfy their constituents if they are to remain in leadership positions after the next election. Thus, the stage is set for highly disruptive relations and even a lengthy strike, because neither side is willing (or politically able) to temper its stand. Cooperation is diminished; anxiety and animosity make the work environment considerably less pleasant.

Collective action imposes new responsibilities on members. Besides dues that have to be paid by all members, someone must assume the leadership role. Others must facilitate the functioning of the union by assuming roles on negotiations and grievance committees. Still others must act as stewards to help members process complaints through the preliminary stages of the grievance procedure. This work takes time and effort for which there are few tangible rewards. In fact, seldom do these roles pay more than out-of-pocket expenses, and sometimes they do not even cover that.

PROFESSIONAL IMPLICATIONS

Professionals have not shown much interest in collective action. Some view it as unprofessional; others see their allegiance as being to the profession and not to a particular job or employer. Since the role of the professional is different from that of other health care employees, the implications of collective action for this group merit a separate examination.

Besides the advantages and disadvantages afforded other health care workers, professionals have some unique concerns. One important issue is the question of professionalism and collective action: are the two compatible? Again the answer depends upon each individual's assessment of the trade-offs involved.

Benefits

Collective action provides the professional with an opportunity to influence the methods and quality of services rendered. Bargaining can establish a partnership between the desires of the manager of the facility and the judgment of the professional. Without an employee organization professionals must rely solely upon the discretion of the administrators. This benefit therefore is of value only in the face of unresponsive management [8].

Although health care facilities historically have paid low wages, nowhere is this problem more obvious than among professionals. In most communities it is common for skilled tradespeople to earn more than health care professionals — other than physicians and administrators. Public reaction may be one of outrage over the inflationary impact of more realistic salaries to professionals. Nevertheless collective action does offer a vehicle through which long-standing inequities in pay can be lessened.

Through a strong, economically-oriented organization the stature of the various professions in health care can be enhanced. Most professional associations exist to further the standards of the profession and provide continuing education for the members. A labor organization can carry on these functions, too. Moreover, since the union represents the professional to the employer and the public, the professional associations that fail to grapple with collective action may be replaced by unions. Restated, labor organizations have the *potential* to serve the multiple needs of today's professionals. Whether that potential will be realized or whether professional associations will actively represent their members through collective bargaining is yet to be determined.

Shortcomings

The single most recurrent argument against collective action for professionals is that it is unprofessional to belong to a union. Practitioners are forced to relinquish their individuality to the majority wishes of the group. If the labor organization negotiates a requirement that applies to all members of a particular professional classification, and a minority of members disagree, they must accede to the wishes of the majority. Although this is an important consideration for many professionals, it also arises in any situation in which the administration passes a rule that applies to all professionals.

An extension of the unprofessional thesis is the widespread feeling that joining a union is demeaning. Labor organizations, in the minds of many, are for unskilled or skilled workers, not professionals. If union activity becomes common, some feel the status of the profession may be diminished in the eyes of the public. The rapid acceptance of collective action by teachers, physicians, and other professionals, however, is slowly making the public realize that unionization does not mean less dedication or less professionalism.

Many health care professionals are in a staff or advisory role. Although they have much responsibility, few have had authority. In addition many are women. These two observations together present an unusual shortcoming. First, since so few professionals have had experience with positions of authority, capable leadership will take time to emerge.

Second, the leadership question is particularly acute among groups dominated by women — nurses, nutritionists, and so forth. Many women have viewed their employment as a job rather than a career. As a result a smaller percentage of the members have shown an interest in seeking leadership positions. Current societal trends and the number of women heads of households, however, indicate that the traditional role of women is rapidly changing. As more of them become career oriented, an increasing number of capable leaders will emerge [6].

One last shortcoming is the effect of collective action on managers who are also members of a professional association. If the bargaining group and the professional association are one and the same, top administration may require professionals (who are also supervisors) to forego membership in the professional association. Since government regulations and the employer's need for solidarity among administrators preclude membership in the labor organization, this may mean the loss of professional affiliations for professionals who are in management positions. This issue may not be resolved for years. At present professional groups are establishing two separate entities within their associations: one for collective action and one for professional education or advancement. These actions are an attempt to satisfy administrative and government decision-makers. If such arrangements are accepted, this particular disadvantage of unions to professionals will be overcome.

SUMMARY

The motivations that lead people to join or not join unions are diverse. The major determinant of these motivations is management. Administrators who are not attuned to the needs of workers or who misuse their power stimulate employee interest in labor organizations. The response of administrators to unions includes an increased centralization of decisions affecting workers. This minimizes legal complications and assures uniformity of treatment. First-level supervisors — usually the weakest link in management's resistance to unions — become the object of increased attention primarily in the form of training.

The advantages and disadvantages of collective bargaining are the crucial points to consider for those involved in union activity. The major advantages to employees are an equalization of power and control over

1aking process. Strikes and the formalization of an adversary
ip between administrators and subordinates are the primary
~~uisaavant~~ages.
Professionals have to evaluate collective action within the context
of their unique status. The principal advantage is greater influence in
the design and delivery of health care. The stigma of unprofessionalism
attached to unions by some is a major deterrent to membership.

In the assessment of collective action the means and ends sought by
labor organizations and administrators provide an insight into the roles
played by both parties. Regardless of the conclusions arrived at by
administrators or professionals, there are governmentally imposed constraints. These regulations control the actions of all providers in health
care facilities. Embodied in the Labor Management Relations Act, as
amended, is a mixture of rights and prohibitions. A review of these
in the next chapter and of their enforcement procedures in Chapter 5
will explain the government's role.

POINTS FOR REFLECTION

1. Why do people join or not join unions?
2. What are likely administrative responses to the threat of unionization?
3. What are the issues that confront a professional in evaluating the
   appropriateness of joining a union?
4. What are the advantages and disadvantages to joining a union?

SELECTED READINGS

1. Bakke, E. Wight. Why workers join unions. *Personnel* 22:2, 1945.
2. Deloughery, Grace L., and Kristine M. Gebbie. *Political Dynamics:
   Impact on Nurses and Nursing.* St. Louis: C. V. Mosby Company, 1975.
3. Jennings, Ken. Foreman's views of their involvement with the union
   steward in the grievance process. *Labor Law Journal* 25:540, 1974.
4. Kircher, William L. The new challenges to organizing. *American
   Federationist* 73:1, 1966.
5. Lewis, Robert. The law and strategy of dealing with union organizing
   campaigns. *Labor Law Journal* 25:31, 1974.
6. Parrish, John B. Women in professional training. *Monthly Labor
   Review* 97:40, 1974.

7. Raphael, Edna E. Working women and their membership in labor unions. *Monthly Labor Review* 97:27, 1974.
8. Weatherbee, Robert N. "Nurses and Collective Bargaining in The Bay Area." Master of Business Administration Thesis, Berkeley, University of California, 1968.

4

Government Goals and Constraints

Ignorance of the law excuses no man.
  — John Selden

The actions of employers and unions hold implications for all of society. Nowhere is this more obvious than in the health care delivery system. The wages demanded by unions, the willingness and ability of health care institutions to meet those demands, and the ramifications of their decision on the cost and quality of health care affect the well-being of every community.

Whenever citizens are subject to the decisions made by organizations, politicians at every level of government become interested. This interest is followed by laws to protect society from the decision-makers' actions if there is a possibility that third parties (the public) may he harmed. The potential for damage is so great that employment-related legislation has proliferated [4]. There have been laws passed to establish minimum wages under the Fair Labor Standards Act (1938), to guarantee most workers a modest pension through the Social Security Act (1935), to lessen discrimination in employment via the Civil Rights Act (1964), and to assure safe working conditions with the Occupational Safety and Health Act (1970).

To minimize disruption to the economy from labor-management disputes, Congress enacted the National Labor Relations Act (NLRA) in 1935. In 1947 Congress amended this law by making it a part of the Labor Management Relations Act. The resulting body of law—which can correctly be referred to as either the National Labor Relations Act (NLRA) or the Labor Management Relations Act (LMRA)—was further amended in 1959 and 1974. The NLRA and its subsequent amendments constitute the major restrictions upon the actions of unions and employers.

These constraints are given a broad interpretation by the government agency that was established to enforce the law — the National Labor Relations Board (NLRB). Through the NLRB's rulings, these acts have been given considerable force in shaping the relationship between unions, employers, and employees. To understand the role of the NLRB, however, it is necessary to examine the purpose and constraints behind the National Labor Relations Act as it has been amended. This important law will be explained in this chapter, and the next chapter will explore the policies and procedures of the National Labor Relations Board.

LABOR LEGISLATION

In the United States the actions of the government are invalid unless permitted by the Constitution. In other words it is the Constitution that gives the government the power to regulate the actions of its citizens.

The power to regulate health care employers and unions comes from Section VIII of the United States Constitution. This provision gives Congress the right to regulate commerce between the states. This power applies to health care institutions because they purchase goods and services through interstate commerce.

By applying this constitutional power Congress was able to achieve two goals: First, disruption of the health care industry became subject to federal regulations. Second, rights previously denied health care workers were extended to these employees.

Restraints on Health Care Workers

Obviously the concern of Congress was not the disruption of interstate commerce by strikes in the health field. If Exxon or General Motors were closed by a strike, the repercussions throughout the economy would be grave. But a strike against one hospital, or even a chain of hospitals, does not materially interfere with the flow of commerce in the United States. What it does do is jeopardize the well-being of clients in health care institutions.

Rather than implement a no-strike law with all its negative political ramifications, Congress brought nonprofit health care institutions under the coverage of the Labor Management Relations Act (i.e., National Labor Relations Act, as amended). This does not eliminate the possibility of strikes, but provisions in the act require lengthy notification procedures and allow time for alternative patient care arrangements to be made. Before this legislation, strikes could occur without preliminary and enforceable notification procedures. Now the National Labor Relations Board (NLRB) can intercede against either administrators or associations when the notification process is not followed. A group that does not adhere to the notification requirements can be prosecuted.

New Rights of Health Care Workers

Health care workers are now entitled to all rights granted by the 1935 NLRA. Section 7 of the NLRA enumerates federally protected rights that employers and labor organizations *must* honor. If any point in section 7 is violated, the aggrieved employee can obtain redress from the wrongdoer through the federal government and at the government's expense. The rights of employees as stated in section 7 are as follows:

Employees shall have the right to selforganization, to form, join, or assist labor organizations, to bargain collectively through representatives of their own choosing, and to engage in other concerted activities for the purpose of collective bargaining or other mutual aid or protection, and shall also have the right to refrain from any or all of such activities except to the extent that such right may be affected by an agreement requiring membership in a labor organization as a condition of employment as authorized in section 8 (a) (3).

In other words, the goal of the NLRA is to give workers the right to become involved in all phases of collective action. This includes the right to form, join, or assist others in establishing a labor organization. Through representatives of the employees' choosing, personnel covered by the NLRA can bargain with the employer. "Concerted activities," such as strikes, are permitted for the purpose of pursuing collective bargaining aims or for mutual protection [2]. Moreover the employee has the right *not* to do any of these things. Each person is free to decide for himself or herself.

The only exception contained in section 7 arises when the labor organization and the employer have negotiated a union shop clause into the contract. As explained in Chapter 3, the union shop clause typically states that all persons who work for a particular employer and are eligible for membership in the employee organization must join the organization within a specified period of time, usually thirty days. If a person is fired under a valid union shop clause for failure to join or to pay dues, the discharge is legal, and the government does not become involved. (When the LMRA was passed in 1947 to amend the NLRA, Congress let each state decide whether union shop provisions would be permissible.)

Prohibitions on Management

In the absence of a law regulating management's actions it would be virtually impossible for workers to form a union. Administrators could discriminate in hiring or tenure on the basis of each worker's prounion or antiunion sympathies. Prior to the 1930's it was common practice to have contracts with clauses stating that union involvement by the employee was grounds for discharge. Although these *yellow-dog* contracts (as they were called) are now illegal, many people still believe that union activity is a fast way to get fired. The discharge of a worker covered by the NLRA is against the law. Where it is proved that the motivation for termination is an employee's union activities, reinstatement with back pay follows.

The federal laws limiting management actions offset management's power. Were there no restraints on administrative power, the rights in section 7 would be meaningless.

Section 8 (a)

The major limitations imposed upon employers are listed in section 8(a) of the National Labor Relations Act. These prohibitions are called *unfair labor practices* (ULP). When a ULP occurs, the employer is held responsible.

It is through the legal principle of agency that all blame for a management-committed ULP violation falls upon the employer. This legal axiom states that the principal (i.e., the employer) is responsible for the acts of its agents (i.e., top managers, middle-level managers, and first-level supervisors). Thus a hospital administrator may decree that workers will not be discriminated against for union activity. If a supervisor discharges an employee solely for union activity, however, the hospital is held responsible because an agent (the supervisor) of the principal (the employer) broke the law. This is true even though the supervisor's actions were in direct conflict with the desires of top management.

There are five unfair labor practices that employers are prohibited from engaging in. These are *interference,* 8(a)(1); *domination,* 8(a)(2); *discrimination,* 8(a)(3); *discrimination for testimony,* 8(a)(4); and *refusal to bargain,* 8(a)(5).

Interference, 8(a)(1) The most recurrent management violation is interference, or, as it is commonly referred to, an *8(a)(1).* An 8(a)(1) ULP occurs whenever employers (or their agents) "interfere with, restrain, or coerce employees in the exercise of the rights guaranteed in section 7." This is the most common ULP, because whenever another ULP occurs, the employer is usually considered to have also interfered with the worker's section 7 rights. That is, if an employee is discriminated against under an 8(a)(3) ULP, interference with that person's section 7 rights has also occurred. The single charge of interference is possible also. For example, suppose the nonsupervisory registered nurses are forming a collective group to bargain with the management of a hospital. To head off unionization, the administrators decide to raise wages for all RN's by 10 percent. Such a unilateral increase in wages during an organizing drive is seen as interference; the employer is interfering with the nurses' section 7 rights to form a union free of management intervention.

Another typical interference 8(a)(1) violation is for management to express coercive opinions. If in the previous example the director of nursing (a member of management) stated, "Anyone who joins the association will be fired," then the nurses could charge the hospital with an 8(a)(1) violation. The director is interfering with the NLRA section 7 rights of the nonsupervisory nurses.

Circulation of antiunion petitions is done to weaken an organizing or already organized employee group. These petitions are legal if drafted and circulated by employees. If initiated or actively supported by members of management, however, such petitions are an 8(a)(1) unfair labor practice.

It is impracticable to list all the examples of 8(a)(1) interference unfair labor practices; it is improbable anyone could retain them if they were listed. Instead most administrators try to remember a general rule: do not discharge, discipline, or threaten employees because they desire to bargain, organize, or engage with others to aid or protect themselves.

Domination, 8(a)(2) Sometimes employers adopt the strategy, "If you can't beat 'em, join 'em." Rather than trying to stop employees from forming collective bargaining groups, administrators attempt to control the group. This too is a ULP.

In section 8(a)(2) the law states, "It shall be an unfair labor practice for an employer to dominate or interfere with the formation or administration of any labor organization or contribute financial or other support to it...." When management actually controls the employee group, the government — once it has determined domination — usually remedies the situation by forcing the employer to cease dealing with the dominated group. The employees are then free to form a new labor organization. Although the practice of company unions was common in the 1920's and 1930's, intentional and total control over labor organizations by employers is not prevalent today. When it does happen, it is often because the employer is paying all the union's expenses or giving union leaders special compensations that, in the opinion of the government, prevent the union from truly representing the wishes of its members.

Recognizing and dealing with a union that does not represent a majority of the employees is another situation that may lead to a domination 8(a)(2) charge. This too seldom occurs. When it happens, it is usually the result of management's desire to deal with one union rather than with another.

Subtle domination is more typically the problem today. Again numerous examples are available. Some employers, in a sincere attempt to be cooperative (not dominant), have given labor organizations free office space or supplies. Likewise some union leaders have received wages or expenses or both while away from work on union business. These outlays by the employer constitute a minor form of domination. The assistance is not normally viewed as so crucial that the labor organization should be disbanded. The remedy is almost always an NLRB decree telling the employer to cease such activities and desist from them in the future.

The National Labor Relations Act (NLRA) permits leaders and

members of the employee group to confer with the employer during working hours without loss of time or pay. Consulting with management on company time is not considered an 8(a)(2) violation. Managers must be especially careful, however, that in-house employee committees are not considered to be labor organizations dominated by management [11].

The complexities of 8(a)(2) domination charges do not permit a review of every possible violation. Here again a general rule is a more effective guide to management action: the employer should not assist the union with financial or nonfinancial aid.

Discrimination, 8(a)(3) It is an 8(a)(3) ULP for an employer "by discrimination in regard to hire or tenure of employment or any term or condition of employment to encourage or discourage membership in any labor organization. . . ." Except for a valid union shop clause, the employer may not evaluate potential applicants on the basis of union involvement or the lack thereof. Once hired, union members must not be treated differently from nonmembers.

When unfavorable jobs are consistently assigned to members (or non-members), when pay levels are different for the same classification of workers depending on union membership, or when any other differentiation in the rewards or benefits is made because of union involvement, the employer is violating the discrimination provisions of the law. The employer's motivation for differentiation is likely to be very complex; reasons that have nothing to do with discrimination are often present.

When the employer takes action against a union activist, a work-related reason is usually cited. This is called a *dual motive* case, since the employer's motivation may be based on a desire to discriminate or a valid problem with employee performance. Suppose an outspoken employee is actively helping form a labor organization. This same worker has had twelve absences during the previous twelve months, and the personnel policy states that "more than twelve absences within one year is grounds for dismissal." Subsequently this activist is sick and misses a thirteenth day. Management discharges the worker and cites the long-standing absence policy as justification. Has an 8(a)(3) ULP occurred?

There is no simple answer. The NLRB, if notified, will investigate. During the process the agency will try to determine the following points:

1. *Knowledge of union activity.* Did the employer know of the worker's union involvement? If even one supervisor knew, it is considered that the employer knew.
2. *Antiunion background.* Does the organization have a history of antiunion activity? Previous ULP charges against the organization are considered an indication of an antiunion stand.
3. *Unequal enforcement of rules.* Are the rules selectively applied? If other people had thirteen absences within a year and were not discharged, then the employer's case is weakened.
4. *Timing of discipline.* Did the discipline occur at a time when it would be likely to bias other personnel? Discipline, when dual motives are present, is especially suspect just before employees must decide on whether to join a union.
5. *Questioning and surveillance.* Has management questioned or observed eligible union members to determine their interest? Besides often being an ULP in itself, such an action by management can be used to show knowledge of union activity.

The more questions that are answered in the affirmative, the more likely it is that the employer will be found guilty of discrimination, an 8(a)(3) violation. In the example given here, unequal enforcement of the rules is a controlling factor. If other employees have had thirteen or more absences, then the termination of the union activist will be considered a ULP. If all other employees who missed thirteen days have been fired, then the dismissal of the union activist will probably be ruled justifiable. No ULP will be charged.

Management therefore may discipline a worker for *any* reason. If, however, the intent *or* result of the discipline is to encourage or discourage unionism, it is an 8(a)(3) unfair labor practice. The general rule to remember is, do not discipline if the result would be discriminatory. If discipline is rendered, management must be able to back up its decision with evidence. Had management been unable to show the National Labor Relations Board documentation (personnel records) of poor attendance in the above example, the employer would have had no defense.

Discrimination for Testimony, 8(a)(4) To make the administration of the law work, section 8(a)(4) was included. This provision makes it a ULP for an employer "to discharge or otherwise discriminate against an employee because he has filed charges or given testimony under this Act. . . ."

In other words if an individual complains (or supports someone else's complaint) to the NLRB, the employer may not discriminate against that person for complaining. The examples of potential discrimination are the same as those under 8(a)(3) discrimination. There is no question as to whether the employer knows of the testimony, since testimony is given before an administrative law judge with the employer's representatives present.

The general rule is to avoid discrimination against anyone who provides testimony or files charges under the act; or, more simply, to ignore that person's role in the complaint.

Refusal to Bargain, 8(a)(5): Finally it is an unfair labor practice for an employer "to refuse to bargain collectively with the representatives of his employees. . . ."

Probably no employer ULP is harder to comprehend than this one. Even NLRB officials do not uniformly agree upon what is required by 8(a)(5).

In another part of the National Labor Relations Act, section 8(d), Congress stated that bargaining requires the parties "to meet at reasonable times and confer in good faith with respect to wages, hours, and other terms and conditions of employment." The NLRB and court decisions have given this part of 8(d) a broad interpretation.

Though the law says "wages," wages have been interpreted to mean any form of remuneration, including fringe benefits. Employers have had to negotiate over vacations, holidays, merit raises, insurance, retirement, bonuses, overtime, and other items that reward the individual for work. Hours generally mean starting and stopping times, number of hours required per day, rest breaks, lunch breaks, cleanup time, and other issues related to the time of work.

The catchall phrase "other terms and conditions of employment" causes negotiations to cover a wide range of topics. Use of subcontractors, plant rules, productivity of workers, seniority, union security, grievance procedures, safety, and working conditions are topics that employers must negotiate.

The law does provide that neither party is compelled "to agree to a proposal or require the making of a concession." Both sides must bargain in good faith, but the law does not require management to give anything to the union or vice versa. Usually the power of each side is sufficient to win concessions in negotiations, since each party wishes to avoid sanctions by the other.

Besides the obvious ULP of refusing to meet with the employee representative, other employer actions have been held to be 8(a)(5) violations. One of the most prevalent transgressions occurs when an employer takes a unilateral action that affects the wages, hours, or other conditions of employment. A change in pay schedules, the pay date, prices charged in the employer's cafeteria, the amount of cleanup time, and countless other unilateral actions have been ruled ULP's. (Generally these 8(a)(5) charges arise when an employer makes a change in violation of the contract without obtaining the agreement of the union. Mutually agreed upon changes are legally permissible.)

Other 8(a)(5) violations occur when an employer insists on negotiating a topic that is a voluntary issue, such as how much union officers receive from the union to defray expenses. Similarly, if an employer refuses to discuss a topic that is a proper subject for negotiations it is also an 8(a)(5) ULP. Conditions imposed by management before negotiating with the authorized representative of the employees are unfair labor practices under 8(a)(5).

Here again the list of potential 8(a)(5) violations is staggering. The general rule is that management should be willing to negotiate all items concerning wages, hours, and conditions of employment. Furthermore, once negotiated, changes should be made only in consultation with the employees' representatives.

Other Legal Limitations

The 8(a) provisions are the principal labor relations stumbling blocks for employers. The National Labor Relations Act is only one part of the restraints that must be considered, however. Management may not agree to violate the requirements found in other laws such as the Occupational Safety and Health Act (1970), the Civil Rights Act (1964), the Age in Employment Discrimination Act (1967), the Employee Retirement Income Security Act (1974), the Fair Labor Standards Act (1938), and the Social Security Act (1935), to mention just a few.

In addition to other legislation, court and NLRB rulings continue to expand the list of prohibitions. Some examples: health care managers may not question an individual employee alone concerning matters that may lead to discipline, if the worker wants a labor organization representative present. If management makes claims of financial inability to meet union demands, it must document its assertions. The employer must furnish all information required by the labor group to bargain with understanding. (Although confidential material may be withheld, job classifications, position descriptions, present salary information, and the like have been ruled as necessary for the union to represent its members effectively.) Failure to do this can result in charges of interference 8(a)(1) or refusal to bargain 8(a)(5) or both.

These limitations are examples of a constantly evolving body of rules and constraints. New interpretations are made every week. To stay aware of new rulings health care managers should obtain labor law services published by such companies as Commerce Clearing House, Inc., Prentice-Hall, Inc., or the Bureau of National Affairs, Inc. These weekly mailings, along with other newsletters, keep the manager aware of the changing regulations surrounding the labor laws.

Prohibitions on Labor

From 1935 until 1947 no unfair labor practices had been defined as being committed by labor organizations. In 1947 the Labor Management Relations Act amended the National Labor Relations Act and added definitions of seven such practices.

Prior to 1935 managers had power and few limitations. The power was misused, albeit by a minority of employers, and the government acted to limit management's rights. During the 1935 to 1947 period unions had the federally enforced power to organize. Once again power was misused by a minority. Labor organizations refused to bargain in good faith and interfered with the workers' NLRA section 7 rights. To rectify this imbalance of power, section 8(b) was added to the NLRA in the form of the LMRA. Like section 8(a), which lists restrictions against employers and violations committed by them, section 8(b) lists prohibitions against certain activities by the union.

Section 8(b)

The labor organization is held accountable for 8(b) violations in the same manner as the 8(a) provisions are held against the employer under

the legal principle of *agency*. If a steward (the lowest level union official) disobeys an 8(b) restriction, the union is charged.

Interference, 8(b)(1): The first union prohibition, 8(b)(1), is in two
parts, (A) and (B).

The 8(b)(1)(A) provision makes it a ULP for the labor organization
"to restrain or coerce employees in the exercise of the rights guaranteed
in section 7." Violations include the use of violence or threat of violence
to force someone to join a union or sign a petition. Efforts to prevent
eligible employees from voting in an election to determine union status
are also illegal. The 8(b)(1)(A) charge can also result from other 8(b)
violations that interfere with the workers' section 7 rights. The general
rule for union officials is to allow each employee free choice in deciding
whether to support the union. Nothing in 8(b)(1)(A) prevents an employee association from formulating entrance or retention requirements
for members, however.

The second part, 8(b)(1)(B), states that the labor organization may
not "restrain or coerce . . . an employer in the selection of his representatives for the purposes of collective bargaining or the adjustment of
grievances." It is a ULP for a union to refuse to deal with management
because of the individual who is representing the firm. The 8(b)(1)(B)
ULP allows administrators to select whomever they want to represent
them in bargaining or grievance sessions. The appropriate guideline for
labor officials is to negotiate with whoever represents management.

Induced Discrimination, 8(b)(2): The employee organization may
not "cause or attempt to cause an employer to discriminate against an
employee in violation of subsection (a)(3) or to discriminate against an
employee with respect to whom membership . . . has been denied or
terminated on some ground other than his failure to tender the periodic
dues and the initiation fees. . . ." Before this provision was enacted in
1947, unions could pressure a manager to fire a worker the union dis-
liked. The ultimatum faced by a supervisor in that situation was: do as
demanded or face disruption from the union. With 8(b)(2), management
can file a ULP complaint with the NLRB.

The only time a labor organization can legally force the employer
to discharge a worker is for nonpayment of dues or initiation fees under
a valid union shop clause. Otherwise union officials are well advised
not to induce management to commit an 8(a)(3) violation against an
employee.

Refusal to Bargain, 8(b)(3): The requirement to bargain in good faith is imposed on employee organizations through 8(b)(3). The law states, "It shall be an unfair labor practice for a labor organization or its agents . . . to refuse to bargain collectively with an employer. . . ." Section 8(d) requires the employee group (as well as the employer) "to meet at reasonable times and confer in good faith with respect to wages, hours, and other terms and conditions of employment." Refusal to bargain over these topics, unilateral actions that conflict with the contract, and insistence on negotiation of voluntary issues (such as prices charged clients or management promotions) all are 8(b)(3) ULP's. Demands by the labor organization for preconditions to negotiations constitute a failure to bargain in good faith, too. The general rule for employee organizations is to be willing to bargain over wages, hours, and conditions of employment. Once a bargain is struck, unilateral changes should not be undertaken.

Strikes and Boycotts, 8(b)(4): Upon the breakdown of negotiations and with adherence to required notification procedures, an employee organization may strike against its employer. This strike action is a *primary boycott;* the union members are taking direct action against their employer. These are legally protected activities.

Other forms of strikes and boycotts are potentially an 8(b)(4) ULP. Whether an action is illegal or protected depends upon the tactics used in relation to objectives sought by the labor organization. To achieve illegal objectives the union may not

1. Engage in a strike.
2. Induce or encourage others to engage in a strike.
3. Get others to refuse "to use, manufacture, process, transport, or otherwise handle or work on any goods, articles, materials, or commodities or to perform any services."
4. "Threaten, coerce, or restrain any person engaged in commerce or in an industry affecting commerce."

There are four purposes listed in 8(b)(4) that are considered ULP's. The first illegal objective, 8(b)(4)(A), is to force or require an employer or self-employed person to join any labor or employer organization. Prior to passage of this prohibition small employers and self-employed people were occasionally forced to join a union and pay initiation fees and dues. This amounted to a not-so-subtle form of extortion. The alternatives were either join or have the firm's business disrupted. Trucking and baking business were frequently targets. In the health care field small clinics, nursing homes, and professional offices would be likely targets if it were not for this 8(b)(4)(A) prohibition. Part of this same prohibition covers attempts by employee organizations to force an employer to agree to a "hot cargo" clause in the contract. Hot cargo agreements are stipulations whereby the employer ceases to handle, use, sell, transport, or otherwise deal in the products of another employer. These illegal agreements allow employee groups to bring tremendous pressure on other organizations — usually ones with which the union has a dispute. The guiding rule for compliance with 8(b)(4)(A) prohibitions is to avoid pressuring employers into hot cargo agreements or into associations they do not wish to join.

Section 8(a)(4)(B) covers another illegal objective sometimes sought by unions: the secondary boycott. A *secondary boycott* differs from a primary boycott in that it is directed at a customer or supplier of the employer with which the union has a dispute. Picketing activity by the United Farm Workers aimed at grocery stores that handle non-UFW-picked grapes is a recent example of a secondary boycott. The farm workers' dispute was with the growers. But by getting housewives to stop buying grapes at selected stores, the growers found they had to deal with UFW or lose sales. In the health care industry secondary boycotts could be mounted against recalcitrant employers. Particularly susceptible would be small laboratories. A secondary boycott — a violation of 8(b)(4)(B) — occurs whenever an employee organization forces an employer to cease or reduce transactions with some other employer.

Another situation that leads to an 8(b)(4)(B) ULP is when a secondary boycott is used to force an employer to bargain with a labor group that does not represent a majority of the workers. Again the general rule is straightforward: collective employee associations should neither pressure an employer to stop doing business with another organization nor seek to have the employer recognize a bargaining group that does not represent the majority wishes of the employees. If the union does not follow this rule, the employer can request that the NLRB obtain a federal court injunction ordering the union to cease and desist. Moreover requests for injunctive relief under 8(b)(4)(B) are given the NLRB's highest priority.

An 8(b)(4)(C) ULP occurs when an employee group attempts to force an employer to bargain with it for employees already represented by a recognized bargaining agent. If there is uncertainty as to which group · actually does represent the employees, management or either employee group with the support of 30 percent of the workers.can request the NLRB to conduct an election. The best rule for any party to follow in uncertain representation situations is to seek a government-conducted election.

According to 8(b)(4)(D) it is a ULP for an employee group to force "any employer to assign particular work to employees in a particular labor organization . . . rather than to employees in another labor organization." Conflicts emerge when more than one employee group thinks it should be assigned certain work. This is called a *jurisdictional dispute.* Since the assignment by the manager often determines present and future work opportunities, jurisdictional disputes are highly sensitive areas [1]. For example, if nurses' aides are given a particular task, and the licensed practical nurses think it is their duty, the LPN group can complain. If they are not satisfied with the decision, they might strike. If they do strike or use other prohibited tactics to force an employer to assign work, the health care organization can file an 8(b)(4)(D) ULP with the NLRB. If an 8(b)(4)(D) complaint is registered with the NLRB, the parties to the dispute have ten days to produce a solution satisfactory to the NLRB. If no resolution is provided during this ten-day period, the NLRB determines which of the competing groups obtains the work. Although jurisdictional disputes are most common in the construction industry, the best rule for unions *and* managers in the health care field is to work out a solution internally — possibly by making concessions in other areas not related to the dispute. Otherwise all parties are at the mercy of the NLRB decision which, although competent, may not be optimal for those involved.

Section 8(b)(4) contains the most complex definition of union unfair labor practices found in the law. Nothing in 8(b)(4) prohibits workers from honoring legitimate strike lines against other employers by refusing to cross through the pickets [2]. Also 8(b)(4) does not bar informational picketing — picketing carried out to inform the public of complaints or conditions within the employer's organization. *Informational picketing is not intended to, nor does it result in, the disruption of the employer's operation.* The assessment of whether picketing is informational can be made by determining its effect. If it results in some nonemployee's refusal to deliver, pick up, or perform normal services, then the action is not informational picketing and becomes a transgression of 8(b)(4).

Initiation Fees, 8(b)(5): When an employee association charges a discriminatory or excessive initiation fee as a condition of membership under a union shop clause, the union is guilty of an 8(b)(5) ULP. This was once used to keep unions of skilled workers small (and wages high) or to discriminate against minorities. Section 8(b)(5) assures that all workers covered by a union shop clause are equitably assessed. The NLRB "shall consider . . . the practices and customs of labor organizations in the particular industry, and the wages currently paid to the employees affected" to decide if illegal fees are being charged. To avoid 8(b)(5) complaints, the initiation fee should be set at a level commensurate with that in other health care groups and not be raised or lowered on an individual basis.

Featherbedding, 8(b)(6): The law provides that a labor organization may not attempt to cause an employer to pay anything of value for services which are neither performed nor to be performed. This unusual practice, called *featherbedding,* arises when a union demands compensation for its members' services, and the employer either does not want or does not receive these services. For example, if the bargaining representative demanded that three nurses be on duty in the pediatrics ward even though two were sufficient, the subsequent use of the third nurse would be featherbedding. The employer would have to pay for services (of the third nurse) that he did not want and — if the three nurses were doing the work of only two — for services that he did not receive.

This provision is essentially without effect, however. Even if an employer does not desire the work, an 8(b)(6) charge will be dismissed if the employer authorizes and pays for it. Thus, if the third nurse is permitted to work and paid in the pediatrics example, legal interpretations of 8(b)(6) say there is no featherbedding.

Recognition Picketing, 8(b)(7): An employee organization can picket an employer's establishment to get the employer to recognize the employee group. Under special circumstances, however, picketing becomes an 8(b)(7) violation.

Recognition picketing is prohibited where

8(b)(7)(A) the employer has lawfully recognized . . . any other labor organization and a question of representation may not appropriately be raised. . . .
8(b)(7)(B) "within the preceding twelve months a valid election . . . has been conducted. . ."
8(b)(7)(C) "such picketing has been conducted without a petition . . . being filed within a reasonable period of time not to exceed thirty days from the commencement of such picketing. . ."

Picketing for recognition is in conflict with the law, if the employer already has a valid labor organization or an election has been held among the same employees during the previous twelve months. Employee leaders should avoid recognition picketing under these two circumstances. If the members wish to replace their present union, the NLRB has established procedures for doing so. These will be discussed in the next chapter.

Sometimes organizers find it advisable to picket for recognition. This is done primarily to inform employees, management, and other unions of the organizing effort. Such actions are legal. However, before the picketing spans thirty days, a petition signed by at least 30 percent of the proposed members must be submitted to the NLRB. Otherwise the picketing comes in conflict with 8(b)(7)(C).

Nothing in 8(b)(7) precludes informational picketing. Even if it lasts beyond thirty days, it is permitted. If deliveries are interrupted or services by outsiders curtailed, the action ceases to be informational picketing. The labor organization then can expect an 8(b)(7) or an 8(b)(4) — boycotting — ULP, or both, to be filed against it.

Other Legal Limitations

Like management, labor organizations are subject to other laws besides the Labor Management Relations Act. Of these laws Title VII of the 1964 Civil Rights Act is especially relevant. Any employee organization that excludes members because of race, religion, national origins, or sex cannot be declared an official representative of employees by the NLRB. Since these forms of discrimination are against national policy, the NLRB will not extend its power to help such labor organizations.

In section 9(a) of the LMRA the law requires the union to represent all employees in a given unit. This includes those employees who are not in the labor organization. If, for example, all registered nurses are classified together as a bargaining group, each nurse must be represented. The people elected to represent this group must bargain for, and assist with, the complaints of all nurses, even though some nurses did not join the union. This is a common situation. Many times a majority of employees help form a union, even vote for it, but when it comes time to join, they do not do so. The reasons for this behavior range from religious to economic. Nevertheless the union must represent all the employees in a designated group without regard to their membership status.

Labor organization leaders are also bound by the constitution and bylaws of their association. Although these documents vary, contract ratification, election, and other voting procedures must be followed. Violations can result in suits by members against the leaders and investigations by the Secretary of Labor under Title I of the Labor-Management Reporting and Disclosure Act of 1959. (The Title I provisions were discussed in Chapter 2.) Both labor and management are bound by extensive notification procedures prior to a strike. Since these procedures apply when disputes arise from negotiations or grievance handling, they will be explored in Chapter 9.

INTERPRETATION

What gives laws life is interpretation and enforcement. These two functions have been delegated by Congress to the National Labor Relations Board and the courts.

It is the duty of the NLRB to interpret specific actions by employee organizations and health care officials to determine how best to carry out the intent of Congress. To do this effectively, the NLRB has developed election and unfair labor practice procedures. These methods constitute part of the due process of law to which each party is entitled.

Besides well-defined procedures, the NLRB has established precedents that provide guidance to neophyte and seasoned labor relations practitioners. Together the precedents and the procedures make the Labor Management Relations Act, as amended, a viable law — a law that is continuously being refined through new interpretations and improved procedures.

The NLRB system attempts to render justice to all parties, as shown by the interpretations of unfair labor practices presented in this chapter.

The next chapter will describe the vehicle by which justice is rendered — the NLRB and its procedures.

SUMMARY

To control the power of employee organizations and employers, the government has imposed a web of constraints. The nominal purpose of these regulations is to protect the free flow of commerce among the states. The main concern of Congress in extending the LMRA to non-profit health care facilities, however, was to regulate potential disruptions to patient care.

One result of including health care employees in this act has been to provide them with the rights covered in section 7. These collective action rights may not be interfered with by either administrators or unions.

Another outcome has been the limitations imposed by the definitions of unfair labor practices. The law states five broad prohibitions on management. These ULP's or "shall nots" prevent health care administrators from

1. Interfering with workers' section 7 rights.
2. Dominating an employee organization.
3. Discriminating against union members.
4. Discriminating against those who provide testimony under the Act.
5. Refusing to bargain with bona fide employee groups.

Labor organizations are restricted in their actions by seven provisions that prohibit them from

1. Interfering with the employees' section 7 rights or the employer's selection of a representative.
2. Inducing an employer to discriminate against employees illegally.
3. Refusing to bargain with management.
4. Striking and boycotting with illegal objects.
5. Charging excessive or discriminatory initiation fees.
6. Featherbedding (charging the employer for unwanted or unrendered services).
7. Picketing for recognition when such picketing is inappropriate or conducted without timely petitions.

constraints would be useless if it were not for the National
ations Board, which has the power of enforcement. The NLRB
devised guidelines and procedures to ensure that justice is rendered.

POINTS FOR REFLECTION

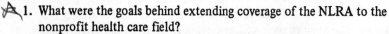

1. What were the goals behind extending coverage of the NLRA to the nonprofit health care field?
2. What are the section 7 rights that health care employees receive from the NLRA?
3. What are two examples of each unfair labor practice on the part of management?
4. What are two examples of each unfair labor practice on the part of labor?
5. What types of strikes are unfair labor practices?   *why?*

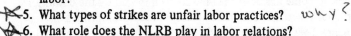

6. What role does the NLRB play in labor relations?

SELECTED READINGS

1. Cabot, Stephen J. How not to get caught in the middle when labor unions start squabbling with each other. *Labor Law Journal* 24:626, 1973.
2. Connolly, Walter B., Jr. Section 7 and sympathy strikes: The respective rights of employers and employees. *Labor Law Journal* 25:760, 1974.
3. Goldberg, Joseph P. Changing policies in public employee labor relations. *Monthly Labor Review* 93:5, 1970.
4. Greenman, Russell L., and Eric J. Schmertz. *Personnel Administration and The Law*. Washington, D.C.: Bureau of National Affairs, Inc., 1972.
5. Morris, Charles J., (Ed.). *The Developing Labor Law*. Washington, D.C.: Bureau of National Affairs, Inc., 1971.
6. Murphy, Edward F. *Management vs. The Union*. New York: Stein and Day Publishers, 1971.
7. Myers, A. Howard. *Labor Law and Legislation* (5th ed.). Dallas: South-Western Publishing Company, 1975.
8. U.S. Department of Labor. *A Layman's Guide to Basic Law Under the National Labor Relations Act*. Washington, D.C.: U.S. Government Printing Office, 1974.

9. Commerce Clearing House, Inc. *Labor Law Course* (22nd ed.). Washington, D.C., 1974.
10. Pointer, D. D. Federal labor law status of the health care delivery system. *Labor Law Journal* 22:278, 1971.
11. Sangerman, Harry. Employee committees: Can they survive under the Taft-Hartley Act? *Labor Law Journal* 24:684, 1973.
12. Taylor, Benjamin J. *Labor Relations Law* (2nd ed.). Englewood Cliffs, N.J.: Prentice-Hall, Inc., 1975.

5

The National Labor Relations Board

That action is best, which procures the greatest happiness for the greatest number.

— *Francis Hutcheson*

No government agency has as powerful an impact upon labor-management relations as the National Labor Relations Board (NLRB). Through its enforcement of the Labor Management Relations Act (LMRA), the NLRB has established procedures and precedents that protect the rights of employers, labor organizations, and employees. This protection of rights results from the twofold statutory purpose of the NLRB:

1. The prevention and remedy of unfair labor practices.
2. The determination of employees' representation wishes through the use of secret-ballot elections.

The NLRB does not actively seek out violators of the act. Instead its investigatory and remedial procedures are activated when an aggrieved party files charges with the agency. The NLRB then pursues the allegations until they are resolved. This is done at no direct expense to the complaining party. Similarly, secret ballot elections are not held until the agency is properly requested to set them up [5].

The NLRB does not extend its protection to all health care organizations. Coverage of an institution by the NLRB depends upon whether the institution meets certain jurisdictional standards. These jurisdictional limitations and the roles played by members of the NLRB will be explained here, as well as the election procedure and the process of investigating unfair labor practices.

JURISDICTION

Coverage under the LMRA by the NLRB hinges upon the definition of three terms: *employer, employee,* and *interstate commerce.* To be within the jurisdiction of the agency an institution must meet the criteria established by these terms.

The term *employer* includes all organizations that affect the flow of interstate commerce except

1. The federal government or any corporation wholly owned by the government or any federal reserve bank.
2. Any state or political subdivision thereof.
3. Employers subject to coverage under the Railway Labor Act.
4. Labor organizations, except insofar as they act as employers.

This means that health care facilities owned by federal, state, or local governments are not covered under this law. Federal employees are given protection by Executive Order 11491 and look to the Federal Labor Relations Council for the administration of these rights [3]. Employees in state and local governments are under the jurisdiction of state and local laws and their corresponding administrative agencies, if any. Health care employees working for railroads or airlines are covered by the Railway Labor Act of 1925, as amended. Finally, people employed in union-owned hospitals, nursing homes, and other health care facilities are extended rights under the NLRA, because the union is functioning as an employer rather than as a bargaining agent in these instances.

The legal definition of *employee* is all persons who work for an employer (as defined by the act) except

1. Agricultural laborers.
2. Persons employed in the domestic service of a family.
3. Persons employed by spouse or parents.
4. Independent contractors.
5. Supervisory employees.
6. Employees subject to the Railway Labor Act.

An example of a provider not covered by the LMRA is a private duty nurse. The private duty nurse hired to care for an ill member of a family is working as an independent contractor employed by the family. If, however, the nurse provides services as an employee of a home health care agency, which under the act is defined as a health care employer, the nurse is considered an employee covered by the act.

An even more significant exclusion is that of employees classified as *supervisors*. In some instances, as in nursing, a clear definition of supervisor has not been made, so there is confusion about who is or is not covered by the act. When employees are clearly supervisory, they are ineligible for protection by the NLRB. They may join unions, but they have no protection against administrative discrimination or reprisals.

The definition of *interstate commerce* as applied to health care facilities relates to specific standards established by the National Labor Relations Board. Realizing that it did not have the resources to extend coverage of the act to every employer-employee relationship, the NLRB established arbitrary cutoffs based upon the dollar volume of transactions conducted by facilities [11]. Whereas the definitions of employer and employee used by the NLRB are derived from the act itself, these dollar-based criteria were administratively determined by the agency [10]. The dollar figure varies by type of enterprise, but for profit and nonprofit hospitals the amount is $250,000. Hospitals (and their employees) doing less than $250,000 of annual gross revenue are not subject to the NLRB's jurisdiction. Proprietary and nonprofit nursing homes, visiting nurses' associations, and related facilities are covered if the gross annual volume of business is at least $100,000. All other health care institutions, whether for profit or not, must do $250,000 a year in gross revenue to merit NLRB involvement.

ORGANIZATION

The National Labor Relations Board is organized in a manner that reflects the duties it undertakes. One set of activities includes conducting elections, investigating unfair labor practice (ULP) violations, and prosecuting wrongdoers. The other set of duties involves hearing cases against alleged violators and offering judicial review. Since this means that one agency investigates, prosecutes, and judges those who commit a ULP, the NLRB is divided into two autonomous offices in order to separate judicial and investigatory functions. These divisions are called the

General Counsel and the *Board*. Each has unique and specific roles in administering the nation's labor laws.

The General Counsel

The office of the General Counsel handles a wide range of responsibilities. It conducts the day-to-day administration of the law, investigates ULP allegations, applies the jurisdictional standards, determines who is eligible to vote in a secret ballot election, decides the outcome of elections, and prosecutes those who violate the law. These activities are accomplished through a network of thirty-one regional offices located in major metropolitan areas around the country.

The organization of the office of the General Counsel can be seen in Figure 4. The General Counsel is appointed for a four-year term by the president and his appointment confirmed by the Congress. The General Counsel is responsible for three major divisions — litigation, administration, and operations.

The Division of Administration is in charge of the staff services that are necessary for most organizations to function — accounting, personnel records, supplies, and so forth. The Division of Litigation handles cases that result in court actions for or against the General Counsel. Typical situations include seeking injunctions against violators of the law and defending cases that have been taken to the federal courts on appeal. To providers, the Division of Operations is the most important component of the Office of the General Counsel, since it and its regional offices enforce the law [4].

In the regional office the most critical role is that of the *Regional Director*. As chief administrator of the regional office, it is the duty of the Director to

1. Issue complaints for violations of the law.
2. Order elections when appropriate.
3. Certify the results of certain elections.
4. Advise the General Counsel.

The staff of the regional offices handles questions about unfair labor practices. When there is a trial for unfair labor practice, a lawyer from the regional office acts as a prosecuting attorney and presents the case

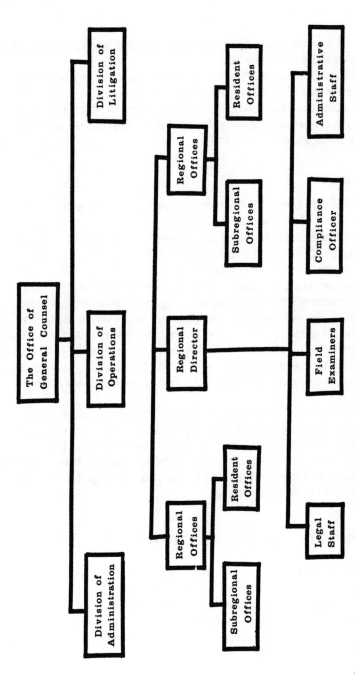

Figure 4 *The General Counsel of the National Labor Relations Board.*

against the wrongdoer. Lawyers may also conduct investigations prior to trials and do legal research.

The other position of immediate importance to health care practitioners is that of field examiner. The field examiner's primary duties are to conduct ULP investigations, supervise secret-ballot elections, and compile the necessary information needed to determine the particulars surrounding elections.

The Board

The Board consists of five members appointed by the president with the consent of Congress for staggered five-year terms. Figure 5 shows the staff that assists the board in operating the office and in reviewing cases. The Division of Information serves as a repository of knowledge that can be drawn upon in preparing and reviewing cases. The Division of Administrative Law Judges, with offices in Washington, D.C., and San Francisco, is responsible for assigning an administrative law judge to hear unfair labor practice cases presented by lawyers in the regional offices. It is one of these judges (in an administrative, rather than a court proceeding) who determines whether the complaint issued by the Regional Director against an alleged wrongdoer is valid. The decisions of administrative law judges can be appealed to the five-person board in Washington, D.C. [7].

The process of resolving unfair labor practices is of concern to all providers, because it is through this procedure that the rights and prohibitions of the nation's labor relations laws are enforced. The systematic method used to resolve a ULP achieves a delicate balance between ensuring the due process rights of the accused while expeditiously upholding the rights of the accuser.

UNFAIR LABOR PRACTICE PROCEDURES

The first step in processing a ULP is for the troubled party to contact a regional office of the General Counsel. (Subregional and resident offices of the General Counsel will accept ULP allegations, too.) Once at a field office the aggrieved will be interviewed by a member of the staff to determine all the pertinent facts. This information includes the

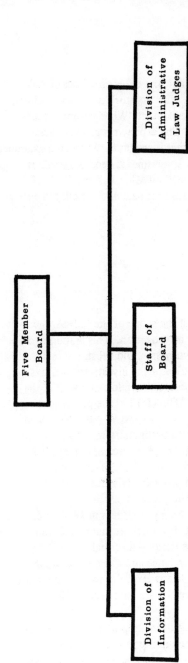

Figure 5   The Board of the National Labor Relations Board.

Five Member Board

Division of Information

Staff of Board

Division of Administrative Law Judges

aggrieved person's name and address, time and dates of supposed violations, names and addresses of witnesses, the violator's name and address,
and a narrative statement from the complainant. When compiled, the
information is reduced to an affidavit. The affidavit is given a docket
(or case) number, and the Regional Director assigns it to the field examiner
or a lawyer to investigate the charges. Sometimes it becomes obvious
during this first step that no violation of the LMRA has occurred. If
there has been no ULP, the entire issue is dropped, and the alleged wrongdoer is not informed of the allegations.

Investigation

Assuming that the charges are within the scope of the LMRA, the
field examiner or the lawyer begins an investigation. This amounts to
verifying the narrative, checking with witnesses, and substantiating the
charges. The accused party is also notified of the investigation and is
asked to submit any relevant information to the field examiner. If the
affidavit is unsupportable, the Regional Director has the power to dis-
miss the charges at this point.

Should the affidavit be supported by a preliminary investigation, the
accused party is requested to submit any further information available.
Cooperation by the accused is optional at this point. If the accused
knows the claims are incorrect and can prove the falsehood, however,
submission of proof may quash the entire procedure.

When there is no information forthcoming, or if it is inconclusive,
the next step is an informal hearing. (If it is obvious that a violation
has occurred — i.e., if a *prima facie* case exists — a formal complaint
may be issued without a hearing.) Attendance and submission of information is wholly voluntary. If innocent, however, the accused is usually
best advised to stop the process by attending the informal hearing and
setting the record straight.

The affidavit and the investigation result in a report to the Regional
Director. On the basis of the information in the report and his own
judgment, The Director will decide whether the charge should become
a formal complaint.

Complaint

Once a formal complaint is issued, the matter becomes one of the United States government versus the accused. The complaint sets forth the charges, which are a violation of federal law. The original complainant has no say in the final disposition other than through testimony. At this point the alleged violator has three options. A plea of guilty can be entered. If this happens, the Regional Director will determine what penalty or actions must be undertaken to "undo" the wrong. The second alternative is not to respond to the complaint, and, by doing nothing, to be assumed guilty. Although the accused, if innocent, finds this option unpalatable, it may be the best alternative. If an employer is required to reinstate a worker and give back pay, this may be several thousand dollars cheaper than legal fees, costs of witnesses, and the general disruption caused by attending a hearing. The third option is to defend against the complaint.

Hearing

The decision to defend against the complaint means an administrative hearing. An administrative law judge will be scheduled to come from Washington, D.C., or San Francisco to the nearest office of the General Counsel, usually a regional office. Although this hearing takes place rather quickly after a decision to defend (normally a month or two), the defendant is permitted sufficient time to prepare a defense.

The hearing itself is like that of a courtroom proceeding. The government and defendant may both introduce exhibits, evidence, and witnesses; make opening and closing statements; cross-examine witnesses brought by each party; and submit written briefs to the administrative law judge after the transcript of the proceedings is evaluated. The administrative law judge will then render a decision several weeks to months after the hearing. Thereafter an officer in the regional office follows up on the decision to assure compliance in the event the defendant loses.

Up to this point the process is expeditious. It takes an average of eleven months from the initial allegations to an administrative law judge's decision. Delays, which can run several years, usually occur when an appeal is made.

Appeals

The Constitution of the United States guarantees every party due process of law. This entitles the defendant to a review of the administrative law judge's decision. The first step in the appeals process is an examination of the judge's decision by the Board. Each case brought before the Board is generally ruled upon by at least three of the five members; majority vote decides the case. The Board may uphold, reverse, or modify the decision of the law judge. In most cases the administrative law judge is upheld.

The next appeals step is the United States Appeals Court. Historically the Appeals Court has supported the actions of the Board in a majority of cases. Should the defendant still be anxious to appeal, the United States Supreme Court is the last step. Appeal to this court is not automatic; due process is complete when the appeals court renders its verdict. The Supreme Court will take only those cases that it feels are significant.

Remedies

Once the appeals process is exhausted, the defendant must comply with the final decision. The remedies applied by the NLRB depend upon the violation. The general theory is to restore the aggrieved party to the position that would have existed had there been no violation of the law.

In the case of an illegally fired worker remedies may mean reinstatement with full back pay and no loss of benefits or seniority [13]. In a case of interference or domination, the correction is usually a simple cease-and-desist order that directs the wrongdoer to stop the illegal acts. When either side has been found guilty of a refusal to bargain, the remedy is a directive from the Board to bargain in good faith (though the Board is powerless to compel one side to make or accept a concession).

If illegal picketing is found, the employee organization guilty of it will be required to cease such efforts. Illegal secondary boycotts are also stopped by a cease-and-desist order.

Whenever there is a refusal to comply with an NLRB directive, the Division of Litigation can secure a court order or injunction against the recalcitrant party. Failure to comply with such a court order can result in a summary judgment that will put the party in contempt of court. Fines (or even prison sentences) result from contempt of court charges.

Thus the ULP procedures provide due process of law for all parties and result in a resolution of the conflict between the accused and the accuser.

ELECTION PROCEDURES

The NLRB election procedures are fast, but they still provide an opportunity for each party to be heard [12]. From the time that an election is requested until the time that it is concluded is an average of forty-five days. Within that time period an employer and an employee group (or groups) are given an opportunity to argue about whether the health care facility is covered under the act, who shall be eligible to vote, and other pertinent matters.

Requirements

The NLRB does not start an election procedure until asked to do so by some concerned party. Usually the election process is initiated by the employees or an involved labor organization. When confronted with a demand for bargaining by someone or some group claiming to represent the employees, the employer is obligated to bargain by Section 8(a)(5) and should negotiate in good faith. If, however, the employer has a reasonable doubt as to whether the claimant actually represents the majority of the employees, management may also request the Regional Director to conduct an election.

An employee demand for an election must be backed up by a petition or cards signed by 30 percent of the employees in the proposed bargaining group. Generally a petition is not filed until at least 50 percent of the people in the proposed bargaining group — called a *bargaining unit* — have signed up. The NLRB sets 30 percent as the minimum figure because the government needs only a "substantial showing of interest." Most organizers realize that if they cannot get at least 50 percent of the workers to express a desire for an election, it is improbable that they will receive the votes necessary to become the bargaining representative.

Hearing

A preliminary hearing is held to assure that all interested parties have an opportunity to voice their opinions. The purpose of the hearing is to determine whether the employer is under the jurisdiction of the NLRB. If the definitions of "employee," "employer," and "interstate commerce" meet established criteria, the regional director orders that an election be held. If, however, the criteria are not met, or there has been an election among the same group of employees in the last twelve months, or the employees are already represented by a bona fide labor organization, the director will refuse to conduct an election.

The date, hours, and place of the election are also decided at the hearing. Election voting typically takes place on the employer's premises during working hours about a month following the hearing. This guarantees that everyone is able to vote and that both sides have sufficient time to present their cases to the workers.

Participation in an election is determined by a given payroll period of eligibility and membership in the bargaining unit. That is, all people in the bargaining unit who were on the employer's payroll at some specified recent time in the past may vote. This approach prevents the hiring of personnel just to vote in the election.

Determination of Bargaining Unit

In the congressional testimony surrounding the passage of the Nonprofit Health Care Amendments to the LMRA, concern was expressed about the possible proliferation of bargaining units in health care facilities. Some legislators feared that a hospital or nursing home might have a number of unions representing different factions of employees. This would result in separate negotiations and labor contracts for each group. The resulting potential for disruption of health care delivery would be substantial.

In an attempt to avoid disruption two questions were considered: First, what groups of employees should constitute bargaining units? Second, within each bargaining unit who should be eligible for membership?

Appropriate Groupings

The congressional mandate made it clear that the number of bargaining units within each health care facility was to be held to a minimum. The NLRB was left with the determination of this minimum number.

In a group of eight cases decided by the five-member Board the following types of employees were held to be appropriate bargaining units:

1. *Technical employees:* workers who are required to be licensed or registered by the state and have undergone some form of advanced or technical training. Licensed practical nurses, x-ray technicians, certified surgical technicians, and others who are not professionals but must exercise independent judgement are in this category.
2. *Service and maintenance employees:* ward clerks; supply clerks; aides in nursing, surgery, therapy, and anesthesia; employees in house-keeping, kitchen, laundry, and printing; and others who do not perform clerical duties related to the organization's business office and are not professional or technical employees.
3. *Business office clerical employees:* billing clerks, cashiers, patient accounting clerks, receptionists, admissions clerks, switchboard operators, and others whose duties are more closely related to the business of the organization than to direct or indirect patient care.
4. *Professional employees:* registered nurses, graduate nurses, and others defined by the LMRA as professional employees. Since registered and graduate nurses are recognized as having a special community of interest, however, they may request a unit separate from all other professional employees.

The determination of a professional is set forth in the Labor Management Relations Act, which recognizes that professionals have a community of interest that may be substantially different from that of other workers. By statute, therefore, professionals are permitted their own bargaining unit separate from that of other employees.

According to Section 2 of the Labor Management Relations Act, the term *professional employee* means

(a) any employee engaged in work (i) predominantly intellectual and varied in character as opposed to routine mental, manual, mechanical, or physical work; (ii) involving the consistent exercise of discretion and judgment in its performance; (iii) of such a character that the output produced or the result accomplished cannot be standardized in relation to a given period of time; (iv) requiring knowledge of an advanced type in a field of science or learning customarily acquired by a prolonged course of specialized intellectual instruction and study in an institution of higher learning or a hospital, as distinguished from a general academic education or from an apprenticeship or from training in the performance of routine mental, manual, or physical processes; or

(b) any employee, who (i) has completed the courses of specialized intellectual instruction and study described in clause (iv) of paragraph (a), and (ii) is performing related work under the supervision of a professional person to qualify himself to become a professional employee as defined in paragraph (a).

A perplexing issue in the health care field has been the categorization of registered nurses and graduate nurses (those who have not yet qualified as registered nurses). Obviously they fulfill the criteria defining a professional. Additionally they display a unique community of interest. State laws stipulating requirements for qualifying as a registered nurse underscore the unique role of the nurse. Some state labor laws even require that nurses be represented by separate bargaining units. This past history, together with legal briefs submitted to the NLRB by the California Nurses Association, the American Nurses' Association, and others, has led the board to permit nurses to form bargaining units separate from other professionals, when nurses so request.

Inclusions and Exclusions

The second phase of bargaining unit determination is the assessment of the eligibility of employees to belong to one of the groupings. To illustrate, the director of nursing is usually a registered nurse and therefore would appropriately belong to the professional category. Since the director of nursing is a member of management, however, this individual is excluded from the bargaining unit and is not permitted a vote in an NLRB election.

The Regional Director excludes from voting and membership in the bargaining unit

1. *Supervisory employees:* those employees who have the authority to resolve employee complaints, make effective recommendations in such cases, hire, fire, or direct others.
2. *Stockholders:* employees who are both stockholders and members of the board of directors of a facility in proprietary (profit-making) organizations.
3. *Confidential employees:* workers who assist in the formulation, determination, or administration of the facility's labor relations policies.

This can include secretaries, clerks, and others who have ready access to such information as part of their jobs.

4. *Temporary employees:* personnel hired for a short or temporary duration (e.g., students during summer vacation). (Regular part-time employees, employees on authorized leave, and strikers are *not* excluded per se.)

5. *Security employees:* guards and others that are employed primarily to provide security to the employer's premises, unless they are put in a bargaining unit exclusively for security employees.

6. *Buyers and salespersons:* those responsible for buying supplies or selling the services of an employer. (Although salespersons are not commonly employed in the health care field, purchasing managers or agents are employed in large organizations.) Neither buyers nor salespersons can belong to a protected bargaining unit.

7. *Spouses and children:* In small owner-operated health care institutions, children or the spouse of the employer may be employed. They are excluded from coverage too, irrespective of their duties.

All employees involved in work that affects interstate commerce are eligible to vote in an NLRB representation election, provided they do not fall into an excluded classification. Of those excluded, the largest group is made up of supervisors and other members of management. Congress decided that the potential for a conflict of interest (or at least a lack of a community of interest among management and workers) did not justify management's inclusion.

Charge nurses, nutritional supervisors, and others whose jobs are a blend of supervision, training, and nonsupervisory work fall into an ambiguous category. Whether they are included or excluded is determined on a case-by-case basis by the Regional Director. As health care labor relations matures, additional decisions by the Board will gradually classify positions that contain elements of supervision. Until further clarifications are forthcoming, the exclusions — and the rationale for them — just listed above will continue to serve as the basis for decisions by the regional director.

Preelection Period

Once the bargaining unit and voter eligibility are determined at the preliminary hearing, a period of four to six weeks elapses before the election is held. During this period the employer is required to post NLRB election notices. These notices state the time, date, and place of the election. The posters inform employees of their right to vote and of the protection provided by the government through the NLRB.

Labor and management representatives are permitted to discuss the upcoming election with employees. Noncoercive views may be expressed by both parties [2]. Unilateral changes by management in wages, benefits, hours, or working conditions, designed to influence the outcome of the election, are unfair labor practices [6].

Representation Election

On the day (or days) of the election the field examiner from the NLRB regional office sets up the election machinery and declares a "no electioneering" area around the polling place. Politicking in the prescribed area by either party is an election violation. Eligible employees, as determined by the preelection hearing, cast secret ballots. Representatives from management and from the labor organization are permitted to observe the balloting, and either may challenge voters who are believed to be ineligible. The normal procedure is for the field examiner to allow challenged individuals to vote and to place their ballot in a special envelope. The disposition of such ballots is subsequently determined by the regional director.

Postelection Procedures

Once the balloting is completed, the field examiner returns to the regional office. The ballots are counted, and the challenged votes are temporarily set aside. If the election is close enough to be decided by the challenged ballots, the validity of each is determined and those ruled valid are counted.

The role of the Regional Director in the postelection stages depends on the type of election conducted. The two categories of elections are *stipulated* and *consent*. A stipulated election is one in which one party believes the election should not be held. This normally occurs when management believes it is not under the jurisdiction of the NLRB or when the petition for an election is defective. A consent election is one which both labor and management agree is proper and should be held.

In a consent election the Regional Director must wait for five working days after the conclusion of voting before rendering a decision on the outcome. During this period either side may file protests over the conduct of the election or submit charges that unfair labor practices occurred during the election. If a ULP charge is filed, the ULP procedure is implemented to determine the validity of the allegation. If it is ruled to be a false charge or one that would not have materially affected the election, the director announces the election results. Either the union is certified as the collective bargaining representative of the employees in the bargaining unit, or the election is announced as having indicated that the employer has won. To win, a group must receive 50 percent of the votes cast plus one [1]. That is, the union must obtain a majority of the votes to become the certified collective bargaining representative. This majority criterion is crucial. If most employees do not vote, a minority of the work force can decide the issue. Whether a person is for or against collective bargaining, each individual should cast a vote.

In a stipulated election the Regional Director does not have the authority to decide the outcome. Instead the tabulation of votes is forwarded to the office of the General Counsel in Washington, D.C., along with challenges, complaints, the Regional Director's recommendations, and all other pertinent information. The General Counsel then decides the election.

Appeals

The primary distinction between consent and stipulated elections is the right of appeal. In a consent election the decision of the director is final: At the end of five days a resolution of the election is rendered. In a stipulated election the decision of the General Counsel can be appealed ultimately to the United States Court of Appeals. Many labor law attorneys recommend a stipulated election simply to safeguard access to the appeals procedures. The entire process in a stipulated election can drag on for years, if the results are challenged in the courts.

When allegations of wrongdoing are proved — by the General Counsel, the Regional Director, the ULP procedure, or an admission of guilt — several options are available to the NLRB. One alternative is simply to let the election stand. This is the usual course of events when the charging party has won the election. Even when the charging party has lost, the election results may be accepted because the violation is considered to be minor and not likely to have persuaded the voters one way or the other. If the violation is substantive and could have changed the outcome dramatically, a new election is sometimes ordered, and the entire balloting process is repeated. A third option is to set aside the ballots and order the parties to bargain. This can occur when management has committed a serious violation that has made it impossible for workers to exercise their votes in an uncoercive atmosphere. Such an order is more likely if the labor organization can show that prior to the ULP it had a majority of the employees supporting it. For proof, signatures on *hard authorization cards* are offered by the union. A hard authorization card is one that union organizers have had every interested employee sign. It indicates the employee's desire to have the named labor organiztion be the collective bargaining representative. These hard cards are widely used in place of petitions (or "soft" authorization cards) that simply list signatures of employees who want an election.

Decertification Elections

What if employees no longer want to be represented by their present union? The NLRB has established another election procedure, called a *decertification* election.

A decertification election can be requested by employees once they have the requisite 30 percent show of interest. Management can also request such an election if it has a good faith doubt that the union no longer represents a majority of the employees. Unsolicited statements by workers to members of management are the proof normally required. Under no circumstances should management initiate or support a petition for a decertification election. To do so is considered an interference ULP – an 8(a)(1). Some administrators, when they learn of this procedure, request a decertification election merely to harass the labor organization. Needless to say, in the absence of sound justification for such an election, management's request only leads to hard feelings and disruption within the union. Little is gained, and much can be lost if the union retaliates.

The decertification process is similar to a certification election. Once the show of interest has been filed, a preelection hearing is held to delineate the relevant issues and to decide on voter eligibility. If the labor organization loses the election, management is ordered to cease and desist from negotiating with the union. The employees are then free to seek another union or to abstain from collective action. If the labor organization wins, the previous relationship continues.

A request for a decertification election will not be honored by the NLRB if the labor organization renounces its representation rights. Under these circumstances such an election would be moot.

SUMMARY

The NLRB is the most dominant government agency in labor-management relations. Its purpose is twofold: to prevent and remedy unfair labor practices and to conduct elections to determine the representation wishes of employees.

To accomplish these purposes the NLRB is divided into two organizational components. One part of the NLRB consists of the office of General Counsel. The General Counsel, through its regional offices, is responsible for the day-to-day operations of the NLRB. It conducts elections and prosecutes unfair labor practices. The other organizational division is the five-member Board. The Board is responsible for reviewing cases brought to it on appeal. In deciding cases, it establishes precedents for future decisions. Many of the constraints facing labor organizations and management are not statutory limitations; they are the result of rulings by the board.

The two most important procedures devised by the NLRB are its methods of dealing with unfair labor practices and carrying out elections. Both procedures are designed to deliver a resolution of issues promptly while giving each party recourse to appeals procedures.

POINTS FOR REFLECTION

1. Describe the functions of the office of the General Counsel of the NLRB.
2. What is the role of the five-member board of the NLRB?
3. What and who is under the jurisdiction of the NLRB?
4. What power does the NLRB possess to enforce its decisions?
5. Describe the election procedure set up by the NLRB.
6. Who is classified as a professional?

SELECTED READINGS

1. Chaison, Gary N. Unit size and union success in representation elections. *Monthly Labor Review* 96:51, 1973.
2. Field, Thomas G., Jr. Representation elections, films and free speech. *Labor Law Journal* 25:217, 1974.
3. Frasser, Paul J., Jr. The right to union representation under executive order 11491. *Labor Law Journal* 25:531, 1974.
4. Gabriel, Ronald L. The role of the NLRB General Counsel. *Labor Law Journal* 26:79, 1975.
5. Gomberg, William, and Bernard Somoff. Improving administrative effectiveness of the NLRB. *Labor Law Journal* 34:201, 1973.
6. Hoffman, Robert B. The representational dispute. *Labor Law Journal* 24:323, 1973.
7. Miller, Edward B. The tangled path to an administrative judgeship. *Labor Law Journal* 25:3, 1974.
8. Murphy, Edward F. *Management vs. The Union.* New York: Stein and Day Publishers, 1971.
9. Commerce Clearing House, Inc. *Labor Law Course* (22nd ed). Chicago, 1974.
10. Owsald, Rudy. A voice for hospital workers. *The American Federationist* 82:18, 1975.
11. Silverman, Carl S. The case for the national labor relations board's use of rulemaking in asserting jurisdiction. *Labor Law Journal* 25:607, 1974.
12. Smither, John H. Does the goalpost move when employers kick about union misconduct during elections? *Labor Law Journal* 25:531, 1974.
13. Stephens, Elvis C., and Warren Chaney. A study of the reinstatement remedy under the National Labor Relations Act. *Labor Law Journal* 25:31, 1974.

6

Organizing: Actions and Reactions

Though this be madness, yet there is method in it.
— *William Shakespeare*

Health care administrators are used to limitations on their power. Government regulations, financial constraints, and technology constantly remind the manager of restraints that must be accepted. Administrators devise plans to minimize the negative implications of these universal and unavoidable limitations. Management then uses its power to direct its organizational and human resources toward defined goals, the only significant limitations left being the abilities and motivations of the staff.

When a union organizing drive begins, administrators commonly fear that the union will block their goals. They are afraid that the demands of employee representatives will make the execution of institutional plans more difficult or even impossible. In addition most health care managers sincerely believe they are already doing everything possible to meet employee needs. New programs and benefits, recent raises, and improved working conditions are pointed to as proof of their efforts. Even though subordinates may view management actions as insufficient, health care administrators often feel that they have done their best, given the financial, governmental, and technological limitations they face. Thus, union organizing drives represent both a potential limitation on administrative power and a rejection of past management actions.

This combination of rejection and threat of constraints leads to two responses by administration. Superficially administrators devise a plan, select a leader, and organize the resources necessary to deal with the situation. Less obvious is their commitment to and prevailing attitude of "winning" at almost any cost. Management at all levels becomes involved in resisting the organizational attempt of the workers.

While this is taking place, employees are wondering how management will react. "Will I be fired for participating?" is a question commonly asked by those uninformed about the legal prohibitions against management interference and discrimination. Potential members of the bargaining unit are torn between expressing their opinions and not "rocking the boat." Furthermore supporting management may lead to tremendous peer pressure against an individual, but supporting the union may be contrary to that individual's personal aspirations for a future supervisory or management position. Compounding the employees' uncertainty is general inexperience and ignorance of the union organizing process.

This chapter discusses the activities and procedures that typically surround a union organizing drive. Both employee and employer perspectives are explained to clarify management and worker reactions.

PRESSURES DURING ORGANIZING

During the organizing drive managers and organizers are under pressure to establish a basis for their cases against each other. Both believe they are right. Under such circumstances there is pressure on every decision-maker, in both labor and management, to justify the means used by the ends sought. To minimize overreactions and transgressions of the law, certain assumptions should be made by management and organizers. For management the critical assumptions are as follows:

1. At the conclusion of the organizing drive and regardless of its outcome the good-will of the workers will be necessary for a well-run facility.
2. A labor organization represents another set of constraints on management action, not the end of the health care facility.
3. Any violation of the labor laws that is committed by a representative of management is an unfair labor practice, whether that violation was sanctioned by higher level administrators or not. Moreover, violations may lead to costly ULP charges.
4. Administrative success or failure in an organizing drive depends largely upon actions that were taken by management *before* the organizing drive began.

Once an organizing drive begins, it is too late for the administration to correct inequities. Not only may corrective efforts be ruled an 8(a)(1) interference violation but, they may also, even if legally permissible, give weight to the organizer's arguments that collective action is needed. For example, a previously unscheduled, unilateral wage increase by management during the organizing drive is generally considered interference. The union organizers can point to the raise and claim credit for it. They can say, "If it wasn't for our union activity, the administration would never have given you a raise." The accuracy of the assertion is irrelevant. If the employees believe it, the raise will actually hurt the institution's case — not to mention the legal complications that will certainly ensue.

There are certain assumptions that should also be accepted by the organizers:

1. For successful collective action to continue, the institution cannot be destroyed financially by endless legalities or prolonged work stoppages.
2. Even if the organizing drive ends without the installation of a labor organization to represent the workers, the administration has been made aware of the problems perceived by the employees.
3. Employee organizers can seek another NLRB election among the same workers, provided that the second election is held at least twelve months after the first one. Failure to win one election does not necessarily mean that unionization is forever a dead question among the workers.
4. If the employee organization is certified as the collective bargaining agent, the new found power will be matched with significant responsibilities.

Organizing, if successful for the union, is the first phase of a three-phase process. The second and third components are contract negotiations and contract administration. All that the organizing activity determines is whether the workers will be represented. It is the contract negotiations that determine what new rights, if any, each side will acquire. In turn, the significance of such new rights depends on how the labor-management contract is administered. Although negotiations and contract administration will be discussed in subsequent chapters, it is important to realize at this juncture that organizing is not an end in itself but a means to other ends. Regardless of the immediate pressures surrounding the organizing effort, actions must be tempered by consideration of future negotiation and contract administration, legal entanglements, and operating efficiency [9].

FACTORS LEADING TO ORGANIZING

Besides individual motivations for joining unions (discussed in Chapter 3) several other factors give impetus to employee-organizing drives. Some of these forces are external to the health care facility and beyond the control of administrators, while others are internal and subject to management's control.

External Factors

The most obvious external cause of organizing activity is a change in laws or interpretation of laws. The passage of Public Law 93–360, the Nonprofit Health Care Amendments, caused professional union organizers and health care employees to reconsider the possibility of forming unions in these institutions. Prior to the enactment of this law the formation of employee groups in nonprofit facilities was subject to state laws or management acquiescence. In most situations neither provided much encouragement. Further changes or interpretations in the labor laws may cause other groups in both proprietary and nonprofit health care organizations to become interested in collective action. For example, if a court of record or Congress decides to extend Section 7 rights to managers, a new wave of organizing activity will result.

Another element beyond management control is organizing activity within the community. Publicity generated by organizing drives may cause employees to inquire into the advantages and disadvantages of collective action. For example, efforts by the Alliance for Labor Action (ALA) in Atlanta, Georgia, included massive media and direct mail campaigns. In addition to these union-paid advertisements there was local news coverage. Many workers in the metropolitan area became aware of their rights, and interest in unions was heightened. Likewise, unionization attempts by professional organizers in nonrelated businesses can lead the organizer to solicit others in the community who wish to organize.

Wage and benefit settlements achieved by employee groups are often reported in the news media. Although the employees involved may have gone several years without a meaningful raise, or profits may have been extremely good at the time, workers in health care facilities may not be aware of these variables when they compare their remuneration with that achieved by others. It is difficult to resist thinking. "How come we never get such good raises?" when other employees receive dramatic increases. Sometimes the answer is "Because we don't have a union." There is little administration can do about such unfavorable comparisons.

The health care facility's growth potential is another force that may increase the appeal of an institution as a target for organizing activity. Public relations directors see future growth plans as a vehicle for favorable publicity. In their zeal for recognition they sometimes overlook the fact that a rapidly growing institution — especially in non-right-to-work states — is an extremely attractive organizing target. Management can control the public relations director's zeal, but building permits and construction activity are impossible to conceal for long.

There is little if anything that administrators can do about external forces. Their presence is an indication that union organizing is possible, if not probable. One viable course of action taken by management in many nonunionized institutions is to monitor internal forces carefully.

Internal Factors

The internal forces are those over which management has some control. The most important is the employee. Excessive turnover, high absenteeism rates, and low worker satisfaction are all symptoms of discontent. The institution is susceptible to union organizing in direct relation to the seriousness of the underlying sources of dissatisfaction. If ignored, the discontent will probably grow.

Closely allied to employee factors is the facility's reward structure. Wages, benefits, and privileges must be internally and externally consistent. If these rewards are not commensurate with those found within the community and within the professions used by the facility, the employer is vulnerable to comparisons by organizers. Perhaps even more important is internal consistency among the pay levels of employees. To be viewed as equitable the reward system must be more than rational; it must be subject to employee input and modification through an effective adjustment procedure.

Communications with *all* subordinates is equally crucial. Any sincere attempt to communicate, however, requires an *effective* grievance process. Health care organizations may have internal complaint procedures, but lower level supervisors seldom encourage employees to use them and when they are used, results are usually slow and seldom satisfactory. A meaningful grievance procedure is one promise union organizers can make and deliver. If prior to unionization activities irregular communications were the rule, the necessary expansion of communications during the drive may be used as another example of "Now management cares, because the union is here." To counteract poor communications, employer-established committees of employees are sometimes created. Although an excellent means of developing communications links between management and workers, such committees should be developed with extreme caution. Their existence may be construed as a bargaining unit; the advice of legal counsel should be carefully followed on this issue [12].

Large health care organizations typically possess a competent staff aware of the importance of employee factors, equitable rewards, and good communications. The principal shortcoming in facilities with hundreds of people is the first-level supervisor. If the "boss" is competent, many other shortcomings will be overlooked or at least tolerated. Incompetent supervision, however, exacerbates employee dissatisfaction in other areas. Workers' opinions of the organization are largely determined by the quality of immediate superiors. Management tends to assume that, if supervisors are technically competent, they are also competent managers. As demonstrated in the *Peter Principle* [11], however, technical proficiency does not necessarily mean managerial skill. Not everyone can move from a technical to a managerial role and do it well. Training in human relations and labor relations is a large part of the solution. But in the absence of a grievance process, many supervisory transgressions resulting from managerial incompetence are never realized by top administration. When an organizing drive occurs under such circumstances, it is hard for top management to understand why all the raises, benefits, and the like have not pacified the employees. To the workers the reason is obvious: mistreatment by supervisors.

EARLY INDICATIONS OF ORGANIZING

In the preliminary stages of organizing, employees are uncertain of what will happen [6]. Rather than confront management with their desire for representation, they keep a low profile. The process is kept rather secretive until leaders have organized the drive and it is well under way.

There are indications that may cause perceptive managers to suspect that an organizing drive has begun. Such a conclusion cannot be based upon any one observation. The larger the number of affirmative answers generated by the following questions, the more probable it is that an organizing drive is underway.

1. Do employees seem to have some definite activity during break periods and lunch that differs markedly from past behavior?
2. Do workers cluster around one or two persons during breaks?
3. Do employee conversations seem to stop abruptly or do workers disband at the sight of a supervisor, when previously they would stay and complete their conversation?
4. Have inquiries into employer benefits, personnel manuals, and employee directories increased?
5. Are criticisms of administrative actions increasing appreciably?
6. Are employees seen passing out cards or asking for signatures on petitions?
7. Is anyone passing out prounion handbills?

Open distribution of prounion materials may indicate that the drive is well under way and that leaders are now willing to come "above ground" to interest others. It may also mean that secretive activities have largely failed and that the open distribution of materials is a last attempt to keep the drive alive.

When management does identify unionizing activities, it should not overact. One supervisor observed many of the listed activities and assumed an organization drive had begun. A couple of days after notifying the personnel department, the manager was pleasantly embarrassed when the subordinates presented him with a complete set of fishing gear as a birthday present. The signatures gathered were for a birthday card and the secretive meetings during breaks were to discuss the present and its cost.

If it is apparent that organizing activities are taking place, the supervisor may be tempted to find out the particulars: who, when, where, and why? Asking employees their intentions to join or not join a union has been interpreted as an unfair labor practice by the NLRB. If manage ment knows who is involved in organizing activity, diciplinary action may be misinterpreted and lead to a discrimination violation charge under the LMRA [5]. The best advice for supervisors is to notify the personnel department of any suspicions. Otherwise, supervisory involvement without careful training may only complicate the employer's attempt to resist the union drive.

POSSIBLE ADMINISTRATIVE RESPONSES

Once organization activity is initiated, administrators are limited in their available responses. Fair wages, competitive benefits, good supervision, and a viable grievance procedure will help assure that employee dissatisfactions are minimal. Admittedly there will always be a small cadre of discontented employees who see the employer as unreasonable. If management has judiciously used its power to further the interests of the workers, however, employee support of the union will be meager. The organizing drive will wither before anyone requests an NLRB election.

Whether or not administrators have prepared for the possibility of an employee organizing drive, there are tactics that can be implemented by *management* during an organizing drive. These procedures must be modified to suit each situation; but the suggestions given here represent a distillation of techniques successfully implemented by many enterprises.

Gathering Information

One of management's first steps is to assemble information about the employee organization. If the workers are handling the organizing with no outside assistance, there is little information that is available or useful. When the organization drive is carried out through an already existing union or "professional association," certain background data can help frame management's arguments against unionization.

The basic operating procedures of an existing union are contained in its constitution and bylaws. A national union or association also has a constitution and bylaws that contain limitations and prerogatives of which employees are seldom aware. Of particular importance are trustee provisions, assessments, and dues. The national constitution and bylaws

explain how and when a local official can be replaced by the national
leadership, whether the members think it is appropriate or not. National
associations also receive a percentage of the local dues (or charge the
local a per capita tax), and levy special assessments from time to time.
To many workers this is hard-earned money from which little direct
benefit is received.

Union publications — magazines, newspapers, and special brochures —
offer insight into union goals and techniques. This information can be
supplemented by contacting other facilities that have had experience with
the particular union or professional association during negotiations and
organizing drives. (Many personnel directors are astounded at the volume
of useful information other employers gladly provide for the asking.)
Copies of recent labor-management contracts tell management how their
benefits and wages compare with those found in unionized hospitals,
nursing homes, or other health care facilities.

Comparative Analysis

Either the employee group or management ends up comparing present
wages and benefits with those of a similar unionized facility. These
comparisons can be a powerful tool either for or against management. A
letter or flyer may be distributed showing wages for specific jobs and
major fringe benefits and ending with the single question, "Are you being
treated fairly?"

What makes this method so influential is that it forces the readers to
draw independent conclusions from available facts. This is concrete
proof rather than the unsupported rhetoric commonly associated with
management or union preelection propaganda.

One important consideration for both parties is the absolute accuracy
of the information. A material misrepresentation of facts such as wages,
benefits, or dues can be grounds for nullifying the election — especially
if the information is released just before voting and the other side does
not have an opportunity to refute misinformation. The only uncertainty
surrounding comparative analysis is which party benefits the most from
its distribution?

Critical Precautions

Two considerations should be "drilled" into every manager:

1. Will a contemplated action be ruled an unfair labor practice by the NLRB?
2. Will a planned action give the employee organization additional arguments to justify their claims?

Certain actions may appear to be an effective means of combating the progress of the organizing employee group. Should these actions violate the Labor Management Relations Act, however, the outcome of the election may become of secondary importance compared with the ramifications of the subsequent legal entanglement. No matter what the election results are, an unfair labor practice may cause the election to be set aside or may even result in management's being required to bargain with the union.

Unfair labor practices committed during the election drive present another problem. If either labor or management is charged with a violation, the other side can point to the transgression. The impact on employees is debatable. It is an interesting argument to claim that the opponent is ruthless enough to stoop to breaking the law. The rhetorical question that follows a violation is "Should you vote for those who break federal laws?" It is a difficult question to counteract.

Free Speech

The constitutional rights to free speech prevail during the organizational drive. However, when the employer's agents claim "free speech" to make coercive, incorrect, or discriminatory statements, the NLRB considers such comments to be unfair labor practices [8].

Prepared speeches and written communications should be approved by competent legal counsel before dissemination. Extemporaneous comments should be held to a minimum. Employees' questions to supervisors should be answered, but it is imperative that first-level managers understand the legal implications of their comments. In addition there should be some internal source from which the supervisor can obtain quick and accurate information.

Clearinghouse

To assure that the information available to supervisors and employees is accurate, a communications hot line can be established. The phone number can be made known to management officials and employees. When a question arises, a fast and truthful answer can be obtained through the hot line.

The people staffing the phones must be knowledgeable in personnel policies, benefits, and labor law. Personnel specialists and members of the in-house legal department are likely candidates. These source people should answer questions truthfully. Biased or inaccurate answers only give credibility to the employee organization. The clearinghouse approach has important advantages. It can be used to quash rumors and inaccurate statements. Incorrect and potentially illegal statements by management are minimized, since management can conveniently obtain quick answers to employees' questions. Workers reluctant to reveal their interest in unionization can secure accurate information and remain anonymous. Even more importantly, the clearinghouse demonstrates management's openness. During slack periods the staff of the internal clearinghouse can poll supervisors for additional organizing information. At the same time they can answer questions and remind first-level managers of the hot line.

Centralized Responsibility

Another reaction to the organizing drive is for top administrators to centralize the institution's response to unionization. This means placing the responsibility for management's efforts in one person. If this is done, the individual selected should be given resources and authority commensurate with the responsibility. Top administrators should also realize that, win or lose, the outcome of the organizing drive was largely predetermined by past supervisory actions and facility policies.

THE ORGANIZING PROCESS

There is no one technique or approach to organizing a health care facility, just as there is no standard response by administrators to the organizing drive. Successful organizers do have methods that have proved effective in presenting the union viewpoint. These procedures have been tested by the reality of numerous organization attempts, but they should be modified to fit each situation.

Organizer

Efforts to form an employee organization usually are initiated by the workers. The day of the union organizer who appears in the parking lot, passes out handbills, and wins the hearts and minds of the workers is past — if it ever really existed.

In most circumstances a professional organizer does not become involved until a request for help is received from interested workers. The reason for this lack of initiation by organizers is that they realize how difficult it is to organize a health care facility, or any other organization, without assistance from within the institution. Passing out handbills without internal intelligence is generally fruitless. As stated by George Meany, President of the AFL-CIO:

Despite the well-worn . . . phrase, an organizer does not organize. . . . Now, as in the beginning, the workers must organize themselves. The organizer can serve only as an educator; what he organizes is the thinking of the workers [10].

Employees do not need a union organizer to form a labor organization. An independent, nonaffiliated employee group can be established without any outside assistance [2]. All that is required is a sufficient number of signatures to get an NLRB election. NLRB officials will provide the novice and professional alike with the necessary petitions. What the organizer offers is a depth of experience. Even more importantly, the organizer or other union representatives can assist workers in the next phases of collective action — negotiations and contract administration.

Preliminary Actions

An important first step in the organizing drive is securing information about the health care facility. Financial records available to the public, rosters or directories of eligible employees, and specific arguments for unionization in that institution must be compiled.

Workers sympathetic either to management or to unionization need to be identified. Those who have expressed strong displeasure for management actions are quietly recruited to form an initial core or cell of leaders. Those interested in moving into management positions in the near future or known to have expressed support for the administration are excluded to minimize advance warning to management.

Initial Meeting

At some point those interested in forming an employee organization will hold an initial meeting. This gathering has multiple purposes. Experienced organizers use the meeting to get a general airing of grievances. Not only do these complaints provide potential arguments for unionization, they also identify management strengths and weaknesses. Furthermore the gripes tend to reinforce the need for collective action among those present. The more vocal discussants are also identified as potential leaders in the organizing drive and afterward [4].

At the meeting, government protection for workers is explained to lessen fears of recrimination and discharge. Names of potential members are sought, as are names of people who could serve as internal communications links with other potential members of the bargaining unit. These discussions help the leaders assess the commitment of those people present.

In-House Organizing Committee

The employees establish an organizational structure, just as management centralizes responsibility and creates a structure to resist unionization. Each member of the employees' committee attempts to identify and interest co-workers sympathetic to collective action. As new members join, those who express a strong desire for unionization typically attempt to recruit additional signers of the election petition.

The in-house employee committee monitors management actions in order to determine current issues that can further the arguments for a labor organization. Disciplinary action, discriminatory treatment, or long-standing inequities are the primary items presented to other workers.

Besides intelligence gathering, the committee plans mailings, handbills, open meetings, visits to the homes of potential members difficult to contact at work, and activities designed to increase the visibility of the organizing drive. These "above ground" procedures are reserved until the drive is well under way and the committee deems it appropriate to surface in preparation for an election.

Outside Assistance

The help offered by representatives from the assisting union or professional association will be maintained at a very low profile. Experienced organizers are familiar with management claims of outside interference. To minimize these claims, the in-house committee is kept in the limelight. If administrators claim that outsiders are destroying the cooperative atmosphere of the facility, the in-house committee can merely print handbills listing the in-house committee's members and their tenure with the institution. This makes future administrative assertions questionable and calms the fears of workers about outside manipulation. Even so, different types of assistance are made available to organizing employees by outsiders, some of the more common forms of aid being the following:

1. Training the in-house leaders to respond to general and specific management arguments against unionization.
2. Helping the committee plan meetings and communications.
3. Estimating the likely composition of the bargaining unit in order to determine who should be asked to sign and how many signatures are needed.
4. Providing supplies, printing, facilities, and related support.
5. Filing unfair labor practice charges and election petitions.

Election Preparation

To get an NLRB-conducted election the organizing group must have signatures from a minimum of 30 percent of the proposed bargaining unit. Fifty percent, however, is usually obtained before an election is sought. Once it has signed hard authorization cards from 50 percent of the proposed bargaining unit, the in-house committee can correctly claim to represent the majority wishes of the employees and demand that management bargain with the employees' representatives. The law does not require an election. However, the law does permit management to refuse to bargain if there exists a "good faith" doubt about whether the authorization cards are valid, which of two groups represents the employees, or some other matter [6]. When such a doubt exists, the employer may request an election. Since the labor organization can lose the election because of a massive unfair labor practice by management, most consultants and professional organizers advise the group to confront management first. If the election is lost by the committee, the employee group can charge that its majority was undermined by the illegal management acts, and the NLRB *may* order the employer to negotiate.

In the interim between the request for the election and the date of balloting, the in-house committee actively presents its case to nonsigners and signers alike. Mailings, meetings, posters, handbills, home visits, and peer pressure are used. Meetings may occur several times a day during breaks, lunch hours, and after work.

"Get out the vote" committees are established with carefully prepared rosters listing eligible voters and their probable sentiments. Those sympathetic to collective action are reminded to vote. In the closing days before the election, phone committees may be put to work if it appears the election will be close. To say that election preparations resemble a political campaign in miniature is an increasingly accurate assessment as organizers grow more sophisticated.

The last critical function undertaken immediately before the election is to select and inform polling station representatives. Both management and the prospective employee organizations are permitted to observe the balloting process, challenge ineligible voters, and ensure that illegal politicking does not occur around the voting area. (Of course, no one is allowed to observe how an employee actually votes.)

Professional Associations

Professional associations that evolve into collective bargaining representatives may undergo a slightly different beginning. The process may start as a grass roots movement among a few discontented professionals. Once under way it may use the professional association as a vehicle to organize for collective action. The primary difference, therefore, is that the members are already organized into a structure, leadership has already been determined, and resources are already available.

The multiplicity of employers represented by any one professional association, however, makes the move to organize largely an individual effort at each facility. The professional association acts like other union organizers in that it provides techniques and assistance aimed at convincing nonmembers to join the organizing employees [4]. Legal consultation also can be made available through the professional association. Nevertheless, the creation of a bargaining unit remains essentially the same as the process outlined for more traditional unions, except for the preexisting structure and potentially fast start afforded by the professional association.

AFTER THE ELECTION

The NLRB election procedure concludes with the labor organization either certified as the collective bargaining representative or not certified. Regardless of the final disposition of the election, the facility and the employees continue to provide service.

Unit Denial

If the bargaining unit is denied as a result of the vote tabulation, the union is not permitted to seek certification among the same employees until after a twelve-month moratorium. During the twelve months the employee group can reassess strategy and begin planning for an organizing drive the following year. If the election was lost by a wide margin, such plans may be dreams. On the other hand, a close election indicates a substantial dissatisfaction with the current situation, and a year of careful observation of management practices can uncover arguments for the next attempt at unionization.

For administrators the election results may prove to be a vindication of personnel policies and supervisory behavior. A close election, however, merely provides managers with a one-year reprieve. Every vote for the collective bargaining representative must be considered a dissatisfied employee. In addition all employees are now aware that they have an alternative – unionization.

Administrators desiring to avoid future collective bargaining must assume that each criticism that has been voiced by the employees' committee is a problem needing an immediate solution. Corrective action tends to reconfirm management's claim of concern for the welfare of employees. Inaction is interpreted as indifference – indifference that some will argue should be overcome by a union.

Unit Certification

If the election is won by the employee group, the NLRB will issue a certification to the labor organization as the collective bargaining representative. This requires the union to represent every employee in the bargaining unit, whether or not that person is a member of the union or association. Management must meet with the bargaining representative and begin negotiating a labor agreement that will specify the rights and limitations of administration and employees. Although the laws and their interpretation do not compel management to come to an agreement nor to give concessions to the employee group, certification of the union requires the employer to bargain with the union for at least one year. If during this time management obstructs or delays negotiations, the employee group is free to file a refusal to bargain charge with the NLRB against the employer.

SUMMARY

Union organizing is an experience filled with pressure for all involved. Pressure can lead to panic and legal transgressions that merely compound the complex situation. To avoid the panic sometimes felt by managers and workers, certain assumptions should be accepted. Primary among these is that no matter how important the organizational drive may seem to be, it is of secondary importance when compared with employee and organizational welfare. After the drive, employees and management will have to work together regardless of the outcome.

The success or failure of the organizational drive is determined by management. It is largely predetermined before the drive even begins. If administrators have not satisfied subordinates' needs, claims made by supervisors during the organizational process are likely to fall on deaf ears. On the other hand, if sound grievance procedures, competent supervision, equitable remuneration, and good working conditions are provided, malcontents will have a difficult time convincing the majority to support unionization.

The primary tools available to administrators during an organizational drive are frank and open communication, a comparative analysis of wages and benefits, and the establishment of a clearinghouse hot line through which concerned employees and curious supervisors can obtain accurate information. In addition one individual should be given responsibility *and* authority to conduct management's response to the union drive.

The employees who desire to form a union must develop an in-house

ng committee that can communicate the justification for union-
.... to co-workers. The short-term objective of the drive is to get
signatures on an election petition or authorization cards. Armed with
verifiable support, the committee can request a government election.
During the preelection period the arguments for unionization must be
kept before those eligible to vote. The long-term objective is to negotiate
and administer an equitable labor-management agreement.

If the employee group loses the election, administrators should begin immediately to rectify inequities pointed out during the organization
drive. Otherwise another drive is likely, especially if the first vote was
close. A union victory means that both parties must prepare to negotiate.
Negotiation is the second phase of labor relations. It is the crucial process
by which each side has its rights and limitations specifically defined.

POINTS FOR REFLECTION

1. What prompts collective action within an organization?
2. What pressures exist for management and union in an organizing drive?
3. Describe steps management can take to monitor and counter union
   activity.
4. What strategy and actions are taken by those involved in an employee
   organizing drive?
5. What takes place after an election when: (a) management wins?
   (b) the union wins?

SELECTED READINGS

1. Chaison, Gary N. Unit size and union success in representation
   elections. *Monthly Labor Review* 96:51, 1973.
2. Chaison, Gary N., and William K. Rock. Competition between local
   independent and national unions. *Labor Law Journal* 25:293, 1974.
3. Field, Thomas G., Jr. Representation elections, films and free speech.
   Labor Law Journal 25:217, 1974.
4. Haines, Edward S., and Alan Kistler. The techniques of organizing.
   The American Federationist 74:30, 1967.
5. Hament, Carrol. Are instructions to supervisors to commit unfair
   labor practices unlawful *per se? Labor Law Journal* 26:281, 1975.

6. Hoffman, Robert B. The representational dispute. *Labor Law Journal* 24:323, 1973.
7. Kircher, William L. Labor's approach to the new worker. *The American Federationist* 74:2, 1967.
8. Lewis, Robert. Free speech and property rights reequated: The Supreme Court ascends from Logan valley. *Labor Law Journal* 24:195, 1973.
9. Lewis, Robert. The labor and strategy of dealing with union organizing campaigns. *Labor Law Journal* 25:42, 1974.
10. Meany, George. Organizing – A continuing effort. *The American Federationist* 74:1, 1967.
11. Peter, Lawrence H., and Raymond Hull. *The Peter Principle*. New York: William Morrow and Company, Inc., 1969.
12. Sangerman, Harry. Employee committees: Can they survive under the Taft-Hartley Act? *Labor Law Journal* 24:684, 1973.
13. Zimy, Max. Access of union organizers to private property. *Labor Law Journal* 25:618, 1974.

Negotiation of a Contract

The future is purchased by the present.
    — *Samuel Johnson*

The power relationships within health care institutions are changed once
an employee organization is recognized. Rules and their formulation
are no longer the exclusive prerogative of administrators. A unilateral
power to establish work-place policies is replaced by a process of bilateral
negotiations.

Unlike labor *laws*, which set forth broad regulations within which the
parties must exist, the labor *contract* stipulates the actions of providers
in considerable detail. Wages, hours, working conditions, rights, and
responsibilities are specifically defined even in the most unsophisticated
agreement. These terms, conditions, and constraints are enforceable,
since the document is a legally binding contract.

Given the overwhelming importance of the final contract, it is not
surprising that labor relations specialists devote considerable attention
to preparing for contract negotiations. Experienced union and management negotiators agree that prenegotiation preparation largely determines
success or failure at the bargaining table. Although negotiating techniques
are explained in this chapter, our primary concern is the detailed preparations leading to negotiations. The composition of the labor agreement
is presented first in order to place preparatory efforts in perspective.

DIVISIONS OF THE CONTRACT

There is no ideal contract. Each agreement differs, reflecting the
unique power and economic relationships existing between a given

employee organization and a particular employer. Certain provisions
are common in most contracts, however, even though the wording varies.
The major divisions of a "typical" contract agreement follow.

Preamble

The agreement often begins with a preamble. It states the objectives
of the parties and their mutual pledge of cooperation to further the
objectives of the employer and the employees. In addition it may include any general limitations on management, union leaders, or employees.

Recognition

At or near the beginning of the document there is a statement that ex-
presses the employer's recognition of the union as the sole collective
bargaining representative for specified employees. Any employees excluded from the bargaining unit are also specified.

Union Security

A union security clause is frequently inserted into the contract to
ensure the strength of the labor organization. Basically the clause requires
new workers to become involved with the union in some way. The clause
may simply be a check-off provision, allowing the employer to deduct
dues from the paychecks of employees who authorize the deduction.
This assures the union a steady flow of revenue, since the dues are re-
mitted directly to the union. A stronger security clause is one that requires every new employee to join the employee organization within a
specified time period after being hired, creating a union shop.

Financial Remuneration

One division of the contract concerns financial remuneration. This
includes wages and salaries to be paid and provisions concerning overtime rates, holiday pay, shift differentials, and other forms of income
related to the employees' work. If not stipulated in separate sections of
the agreement, cost of living adjustments, merit increases, longevity

raises, and other financial incentives offered by the employer are also
spelled out in the financial clause.

Nonfinancial Remuneration

Nonfinancial rewards for work are increasing as a major proportion
of total labor costs within health care facilities [12]. To assure a clear
understanding of these fringe benefits, the contract describes different
types of insurance available, retirement programs, employee services
provided by the employer (e.g., free lunches, car pools, free parking),
vacations, holidays, educational assistance programs, and other forms
of nonmonetary compensation.

Seniority

To guarantee fair treatment, employee representatives strive to have
rewards allocated on the basis of seniority and not at management's
discretion. Union negotiators argue that rewards for long service are in
management's interest, too. Management bargainers counter that the
seniority basis limits the organization's ability to reward hard work.
Some sort of a compromise statement is settled upon, typically one
in which ability and seniority are both considered.

Seniority is used in situations other than promotions. Layoffs, re-
calls from layoffs, transfers, access to training programs, and selection
of work schedules are common applications of seniority.

The contract specifies how seniority will be calculated and who is
responsible for the seniority list. Procedures to be followed when senior
employees' jobs are eliminated and senior employees' alternatives under
those circumstances are also defined.

Discipline

Discipline is always a sensitive issue. Administrators must be able
to correct inappropriate actions by subordinates. The union, which
exists in part to protect its members from capricious acts by management,
seeks to have specific infractions and penalties listed. Therefore, a
portion of the contract is devoted to guidelines on discipline. (Disciplinary rules may be covered in the contract by reference to a separate

document explaining violations and penalties.) Although discipline clauses vary, two elements are universal: there is a statement of inappropriate acts and their associated penalties, and there is an explanation of due process.

Grievance Procedures

Whenever discipline or some other management action violates the rights of a union or its members, a grievance can be filed against the employer. The contract specifies how these complaints are to be resolved between the labor organization and the health care administrators. Issues subject to grievance procedures, time limits, restrictions on steward activities in support of grievance handling, and other relevant matters are generally clarified in this section of the labor contract.

Professional Standards

In agreements between professional groups and health care employers a part of the contract may be devoted to explicitly stating codes of conduct or professional standards. This is to ensure that professionals retain certain prerogatives and that these rights are recognized by administrators. A violation of these requirements also permits the employer to take disciplinary action.

Other Provisions

By mutual consent countless other requirements can be included in the contract. Statements concerning leaves of absence, limitations on union activity, training programs, certification criteria, continuing education standards, employee bulletin boards, safety, time off for voting in public elections, and pension plans are common examples.

The mechanics surrounding the existence of the contract also are detailed. They include the date of the contract, its duration, and the circumstances under which the agreement can be reopened for further negotiations. It is increasingly common to see "no lockout" and "no strike" promises in the agreement. A statement is made that the administrators agree not to lock the employees out of the facility in return for the union's promise not to strike for the duration of the contract. This reciprocal arrangement must provide for a means of resolving deadlocks arising over the interpretation of the contract. If questions of interpretation cannot be settled between the parties, the contract usually permits them to submit the issue to an outside neutral called an *arbitrator.*

UNION PREPARATION

The labor-management agreement is a complex document that includes a wide range of topics. Given the importance of the agreement, the need for careful preparation prior to actual negotiations is obvious. Therefore the major preparatory steps undertaken by the union are explained here, followed by a similar explanation of management's prenegotiation efforts.

Information

The foundation of all negotiations is knowledge. For the employee organization, information must be gathered in several crucial areas before demands upon the employer can be formulated. This involves monitoring activities to determine what is potentially feasible. It also involves an evaluation of the long-range goals of the bargaining unit, the objectives of the local or of the district's parent body, and the objectives of the members.

Monitoring Activities

The union leader is elected by the members. This makes the leader a politician. If the official cannot do as good a job for the members as other leaders do for their members, the constituents may vote for a new local president. Therefore it is imperative to union officials that their accomplishments compare favorably with those of other leaders. This requires a careful monitoring of rival union gains in the areas of wages and benefits.

Financial information about the health care facility's operations is also necessary. In proprietary institutions this information is readily available through reports to stockholders. In nonprofit organizations financial data might be acquired through the grapevine when published figures are not obtainable. Typically, this information is secured from those who are friendly to the union and have access to key documents.

The inflation rate is another important item. The increase in the cost of living is one component in determining what the "minimally acceptable raises" should be. To that figure is added an improvement factor designed to increase the real spending power of the union's members. Inflation data is readily available through figures published by the United States Department of Labor.

Long-Range Goals

It is seldom that union bargainers get everything they want in any single contract. Compromises may cause low-priority issues to be dropped. For example, a union may want a retirement plan completely paid for by the employer. To avoid a strike or simply because the employer cannot afford it, the union may compromise on the retirement plan by agreeing that the employees and the employer will each pay half the costs. In subsequent negotiations the union will attempt to secure retirement contributions which require the health care facility to pay a higher and higher percentage of the costs until the union achieves the long-term goal of an employer-paid employee retirement plan.

In preparing for each negotiation the employee representatives decide the priorities of their long-term objectives. These demands are in addition to higher wages and other annual issues.

Goals of the Parent Body

Occasionally the parent body (e.g., a state association or national union) may seek some uniform benefit or contract wording. When this happens, the local bargaining team adds this to its list of demands. For example, in health care many professionals move from one employer to another. To ensure uniformity in fringe benefits and wages, the parent body may strive to have every local or district obtain similar contract terms. Although minor differences exist, uniformity in benefits and wages is practically a reality in some industries as a result of national union goals.

Goals of the Rank and File

The direct wishes of the bargaining unit's members are included in negotiations. In some organizations each member is requested to submit to the steward or some other union official a list of desired changes. Many are trivial — for example, changes in lighting and thermostat settings. These inputs provide the leaders with a sense of what the priorities should be, however. If a majority of the members want another holiday, but few mention improved retirement benefits, the bargainers may focus their demands on holidays and forego an increase in the pension plan.

Assembling Demands

On the basis of a careful monitoring of the economic and organizational environment, long-range objectives, wishes of the parent body, and objectives of the members, the union bargainers are ready to assemble a list of demands. These demands form what is typically called a "bargaining book." The bargaining book contains a list of the targets to be obtained and their associated priorities. Each request lists the rationale behind the objective and includes reasons why the employer should grant it.

Selling Members

Union leaders know that their only real strength is in the solidarity of their members. If the rank and file are severely split over goals, it is difficult to make the threat of a strike credible. Without the threat of a strike, the union is in a weak position at the bargaining table. The leaders therefore try to marshal support from members for the demands.

Selling the Public

When a potential strike would engender public reaction, as is common in the health care field, the leaders of the employee organization must sell the public on the reasonableness of their position. News conferences and even advertisements in the local newspaper can help convince the public of the equity of the union's position. Community pressure brought to bear upon administrators may force the facility to settle at a higher level than it had planned.

Another advantage of this prenegotiation tactic is direct community support in other ways. Some employee organizations have been able to arrange for banks and mortgage companies to agree to delay installment payments or for local grocery stores to sell on credit during the strike. All these actions simply strengthen the ability of the rank and file to withstand the economic vicissitudes of a strike.

Strike Vote

A vote to determine support for a strike is taken at the beginning of negotiations and just before a strike is proposed to occur. The vote at the beginning of negotiations is to show management (via the grapevine) the solidarity of the membership behind the union representatives. Typically this vote is 100 percent in favor of the strike. The vote just before the actual strike is unpredictable. How long the strike is expected to last, each member's current financial situation, and management's last offer influence the vote for a strike and whether the strike occurs [10].

MANAGEMENT PREPARATION

The major difference between union and management preparation for negotiations is one of perspective. The union generally is on the offensive. The employee organization makes most of the demands, and management defends itself against them. Management must also prepare for a potential strike. As with the union, the crucial phase of this prenegotiation activity is acquiring information.

Information

The information gathered should center around the gains made by other employee organizations in the health care industry locally and nationally. Improvements obtained by other unions will serve as a target for the union negotiators to seek.

Union demands can be estimated from several inputs. One obvious source is past requests that were not granted or only partially granted in previous negotiations. A technique of gradual acquisition of goals becomes evident even in areas in which management may have thought employees had obtained their wishes. For example, the union may have obtained a health insurance policy with a maximum limit of $50,000 dollars, as requested, but may seek to raise the maximum in the next negotiations.

Union publications and speeches are a source of information. Astute industrial relations managers constantly read union newspapers, flyers, and publications. Speeches by national leaders and articles by union research staffs offer insight into the union's concerns. Furthermore national and statewide publications offer reliable indications of national or parent body pressures on locals.

Those involved in preparing for negotiations sometimes overlook the most readily available source of data: other managers and staff specialists. First-level supervisors and staff experts are constantly in contact with a wide range of employees. Supervisors can often estimate the major concerns of workers in informal conversations.

The last input is the employer's long-range plans. This information is not widely used because, unlike unions, many labor relations specialists do not develop long-term negotiations targets. If areas of additional administrative freedom can be isolated, however, goals can be established. These targets can then be traded with the union in exchange for benefits sought by the employee representatives. Careful consideration of the rights necessary for effective management must be part of management's informational input [4].

Bargaining Book

With bargaining data assembled, the next step is to develop a bargaining book. Management's bargaining book contains not only demands and their justification but also cost estimates of probable union requests associated with management counterproposals. During bargaining negotiations, union demands (whether expected or not) can be countered with management offers. The financial implications of each administrative counteroffer are already calculated in tables showing the relative cost associated with each incremental increase in wages, health insurance, pensions, holidays, vacations, and other benefits.

At this point management must estimate its maximum outlay, normally expressed in cents per hour. This is determined by calculating the impact of various remuneration levels on the financial condition of the organization. To go beyond this amount would place the enterprise in financial difficulty. Another figure arrived at is the ideal settlement figure. Contrary to what union officials may think, this is probably a reasonable figure. Administrators realize they must offer wages and benefits sufficiently high enough to retain present employees and attract new workers to fill vacancies [5]. A third figure arrived at is the starting offer, which is typically as unrealistically low as the union figure is high. This third amount is merely a talking figure that will be increased in

return for a decrease in demands by the union. The amount finally
agreed upon by both sides is decided in negotiations [1].

Bargaining Team

The bargaining team for management is selected from top administrators within the labor relations department. Unlike the union bargaining team, which consists of elected members, management negotiators can be chosen on the basis of their knowledge and ability. The leader of the management bargaining committee is usually the highest ranking individual in the industrial relations department. Other members usually have expertise in operations or labor relations. Like the union, management retains a lawyer to provide advice and assure that the resulting contract is valid.

Seldom is the organization's top administrator on the bargaining team. The chief officer of the enterprise is probably unskilled in labor negotiations. His absence also allows administrative bargainers to call a temporary adjournment to consult top administration when the union bargainers pose a difficult question. The delay obviously allows management to plan its strategy.

Administrative Approval

Labor relations experts sometimes feel they should have the final say on objectives, methods, and issues of negotiations. Nevertheless the responsibility for the functioning and success of the health care facility belongs to the top administrator, and top management should have the ultimate veto power over the plans of the labor relations experts. Changes suggested by the chief operating officer must be incorporated if the overall policies and objectives of the institution are to be met.

The presentation of recommendations should include a statement of goals to be obtained by the management negotiators. Once the bargaining session is completed, the administrator can compare achieved goals with planned goals. Top management thus maintains some control over the collective bargaining process without becoming intimately involved.

Strike Preparations

Unlike the case with other industries, strikes in the health care field must be preceded by special and elaborate notification procedures. A surprise strike is prohibited by the health care amendments to the NLRA. Thus preparation for a strike is less critical than otherwise might be the case. There are some preliminary steps, however, that can be undertaken to strengthen management's resistance if a strike occurs. Nonperishable supplies should be stocked. During a strike many truckers will honor the picket line and not make deliveries. Alternative health care plans should be made for those clients who are ambulatory. For those who cannot or should not be moved, schedules will have to be devised to allow supervisory personnel to continue health care. New admissions should be delayed or referred to other facilities. Loans, loan repayments, and other financial arrangements should be made well in advance of the strike. Bankers and creditors often become reluctant to extend credit (without a premium) during a labor dispute.

Immediately before the strike it is common for supervisors or other management officials to be told or "accidentally" find out about the strike vote. If it is anything less than a strong majority, management may be able to obtain its ideal settlement figure. When the mood of the rank and file strongly supports a strike, the employer may have to come closer to the maximum figure [10].

NEGOTIATIONS

There are essentially two approaches to labor-management negotiations: all-or-none and item-by-item. The item-by-item approach appeals to many neophyte bargainers, because it gives a sense of progress. As one issue is agreed upon (e.g., vacations) it is considered resolved and no longer open to discussion. The next item is then discussed and resolved. This procedure continues until each subject has been covered. Its major shortcoming is that the parties may make rapid progress until the employer feels there is nothing left to give. At that point important items may still be unresolved, even though there is little room left for haggling. If this technique is employed, minor nonfinancial issues should be settled first, then major financial issues. A deadlock on a minor issue (e.g., pay for voting time) is not likely to lead to a strike. In any event a contract is not obtained until all issues are resolved or dropped.

The all-or-none system is considerably more realistic, because flexibility is retained until a final agreement is reached. As in the item-by-item method, each issue (or group of issues) is discussed and agreed to before others are considered. Since no topic is closed off, however, one side may concede a previous gain in order to obtain a more important goal. The all-or-none approach means, therefore, that no item is finally agreed upon until the entire contract is negotiated. Furthermore combination deals are possible. For example, the union may have fifty or more minor issues concerning repairs to the facilities that annoy employees. Management may offer to solve a specified number of them in return for the union's dropping the rest. Thus the all-or-none approach has the advantage of allowing the most realistic exchange between management and the union.

Subject Areas

The National Labor Relations Board has decreed that all collective bargaining issues fall into three categories: illegal, voluntary, and mandatory. Illegal subjects of bargaining are those that violate the NLRA or other laws. An example of a law violation might be one side's insisting that the other discriminate against an employee because of the worker's sex, race, national origin, or religious background. To do so would violate Title 7 of the 1964 Civil Rights Act, as amended [6]. Similarly a request to discriminate against an individual because of age may be in violation of the Age Discrimination in Employment Act of 1967. Insistence on an illegal subject as a condition of agreement is a refusal to bargain in good faith and therefore is an unfair labor practice.

Voluntary subjects are those that need not be negotiated unless both sides consent to do so. Prices charged clients, dividends, management salaries, union dues, size of the bargaining teams, and other issues have been adjudicated and ruled as voluntary issues.

Mandatory subjects are those that directly or indirectly affect remuneration, hours, or conditions of employment. Through more than four decades of court and NLRB interpretations, remuneration, hours and working conditions have been interpreted in the broadest possible manner. It is not feasible to classify examples according to these three mandatory areas, since there is a high degree of overlap. Holidays, for example, relate to both remuneration and hours of work. A short illustrative list of mandatory topics provides insight into how widely the NLRB and court interpretations have ranged:

Seniority
Grievances
Arbitration
Work schedules
Union security
Vacations and holidays
Raises
Employee insurance plans
Pension plans
Bonuses
Price of meals served in the institution's cafeteria
Subcontracting of work done by employees
Automation
Closing of facilities or departments
Layoffs

To avoid charges of a refusal to bargain in good faith, the employer is required to provide certain information to employee representatives when the data is needed by them to bargain intelligently. If management relies on job descriptions to determine wage rates, the union may demand to see those documents. Financial records must be provided whenever the employer asserts that it cannot afford the union demands. If the employer claims that salary surveys show management's offer is fair, the employer may be obligated to produce those studies. Even employee files may be appropriately requested by the union [8].

Bargaining Techniques

Experienced labor and management bargainers have developed many guidelines to increase their negotiating effectiveness. As is the case with most rules of thumb, they cannot be applied in every situation. Instead careful consideration must be given to their applicability within the context of each bargaining session.

From the union perspective the strategy is to seek more than can be reasonably expected. The union takes the offensive in negotiations. The employee organization makes demands and management defends its position. By starting out high, the union can compromise in exchange for management's concessions. The reciprocal rule for management is to start low and increase the offer in exchange for union concessions. This is a well-established pattern in collective bargaining. If either side started from a realistic position, the action would probably be viewed as a sign of weakness or merely used as a starting point to be made better as negotiations progress. The rule of thumb becomes "Never lay all your cards on the table at once."

A problem with starting from unrealistic positions, however, is that each side is seeking something it really does not want or expect. One management bargainer rather dramatically claimed that the organization could do no better than its first offer. The union believed the story and accepted the meager wage increase immediately. A few months later as employee turnover escalated, the manager was forced to go to the union and suggest that the wage section be renegotiated. The general rule is "Never seek anything you don't want, you may get it."

Contract negotiations are a sensitive issue. The reputations of the bargainers on both sides of the table are at stake. Confidences should never be violated. Boasting to associates or to the local media tends to make the other side adamant in its position. Negotiations should be conducted in private, and confidences should be kept. Violating this rule makes negotiations slower and far less productive.

Another guideline is never to let the bargaining team be bypassed by the other side. If the union discovers that it can bargain to an impasse and then get further concessions from the top administrator, the management bargaining team will be viewed as the first, and not the final, step in negotiations. If management goes around the union committee to bargain directly with the workers, it has committed an unfair labor practice — an 8(a)(5), or a refusal to bargain in good faith.

Along the same lines it is imperative that bargainers never say "no" absolutely, unless their respective organizations will back them up absolutely. Negotiators must learn to say "no" in several different ways. One way means, "Not now, but if you sweeten the offer, maybe yes." Another means, "No, not without major concessions." This semantic juggling is important. If a negotiator cannot develop, through body language and facial expressions, a negative response with several degrees of forcefulness, the opponent will be unable to differentiate between conditional and absolute refusals. Inability to distinguish these degrees can result in insistence on an unobtainable item. When this happens, the probability of a strike — or at least prolonged negotiations — increases.

On a positive note, negotiations should be undertaken with the philosophy that both sides must win. No matter which party has the greater power, each bargainer must leave the negotiations with some victories. If one side is in the stronger position and forces an unsatisfactory settlement, future repercussions may convert the negotiated gains into a hollow victory. An exceptionally high wage settlement by the union, for example, may lead to layoffs. A miserly contract may result in new leadership taking over the employee organization and proving totally inflexible in the next round of negotiations. Both sides must win, since the ramifications of negotiations are *not* over when the agreement is signed. The administration of the contract and the negotiation of the next agreement will reflect the conduct of past negotiations.

Mediation and Conciliation

Bargainers can obtain outside assistance when a deadlock between labor and management occurs or appears imminent. The American Arbitration Association and state mediation and conciliation services are available, but bargainers more commonly rely upon the Federal Mediation and Conciliation Service.

Each of these groups provides mediators who are trained to help the parties reach an accord. Emotions may have caused the bargainers to be angry and unresponsive; the mediator therefore must placate both sides before any attempt at mediation will succeed.

Mediation involves finding compromises. The mediator looks for common ground on which both sides can build. Past progress is pointed to as evidence that each can benefit while making concessions. To add pressure on the parties to mediate, the mediator may indicate that the duration of assistance will terminate by a certain time or date. This carries the implied threat that, if a solution is not found by then, a strike is likely. The mediator is never empowered to impose a solution [3].

Typically the mediator talks with the management and union representatives separately. During these conversations the maximum and minimum positions are outlined. The mediator may find that each party is afraid to make a concession for fear of appearing weak. For example, the union might be demanding an eighty cent increase but would be willing to settle for fifty cents. Management is offering thirty-five cents but would be willing to go as high as fifty-five cents to avoid a strike. Yet neither side is willing to make the first compromise; both sides appear to be deadlocked at eighty and at thirty-five cents, respectively. These separate meetings indicate to the mediator that agreement is at hand if the parties will compromise. The mediator might suggest that management increase its offer by ten cents (to forty-five cents) when the union drops its demand to sixty-five. Then the mediator might suggest to the employee representatives that they offer sixty-five cents when the bargaining reconvenes. If this is agreed on, the parties are brought together again, and each follows the role outlined by the mediator (even though the overlapping solution is never revealed). Now the positions are forty-five and sixty-five cents for management and for the union. The mediator then may turn to management in front of the union and suggest that if management were to go up six cents (to fifty-one) and the union drop twelve cents (to fifty-three) a solution would be near. If this is agreed to, the mediator might suggest the obvious compromise at fifty-two cents.

Unfortunately deadlocks are seldom this simple to resolve. When multiple issues exist, the mediator sometimes suggests trades: the union demand for a new life insurance coverage might be forgotten if management would increase its contribution to health insurance; management might be asked to increase its pay offer by ten cents in exchange for the union's dropping its demand for another holiday.

The major tasks of the mediator are to (1) win the confidence of each side, (2) placate the negotiators and get them all back to the bargaining table, and (3) find reasonable compromises that allow each side to win. Above all else, the mediator must be seen as trustworthy. This means maintaining absolute neutrality and confidentiality.

ENFORCEABILITY OF THE CONTRACT

Once signed by employee and management representatives, the agreement is binding. Generally management negotiators are delegated the authority to sign for and bind the employer. The union representatives present the final solution to the members. The ratification vote — for acceptance or rejection of the offer — dictates whether the union leaders may bind the employee organization. If it is rejected, the bargainers must reassemble and attempt to rearrange the contract in a manner more suitable to the union membership. The proposals are then submitted to another vote of the rank and file. When accepted by both parties, the labor-management agreement becomes an enforceable contract.

The contract can be enforced in three ways. One method is to settle disputes over the operation or interpretation of the contract by a show of power. The union strikes, and management withstands the strike, until some solution is accepted. In the health care field such actions cannot occur until proper and timely notice is served the other side. Then, after a waiting period, a strike can commence. (The notification procedures will be explained in Chapter 9.) Since strikes are complicated and costly to all providers, most contracts contain "no-strike, no-lockout" clauses for the duration of the contract. Thus this alternative may be precluded by the contract itself.

Another solution is to bring a legal suit in a court of jurisdiction for violation of the agreement. Although feasible, this is almost as impractical as a strike. It is time-consuming and expensive. Weeks, months, even years can go past before a final judicial resolution is obtained.

The third and almost universal approach to questions of interpretation is through an in-house grievance procedure. The aggrieved party goes through a detailed process wherein the complaint is discussed between union and management representatives. If agreement is not reached, an outside neutral, or arbitrator, is brought in to hear the issues and render a decision. These grievance and arbitration procedures are discussed in the next chapter.

SUMMARY

Following organization of the employees the next phase of health care labor relations is negotiations. It is through the process of negotiation that each side attempts to limit the power of the other by a contractual agreement.

The most important dimension of bargaining is the preparations that precede actual discussions. Success at the bargaining table is determined by the power of each party and by the prenegotiation preparations. Obtaining information on the status and demands of the other side is the first step. With that information, each side develops its requests and counterproposals.

The power of the union is determined by how successfully it can conduct (or potentially conduct) a strike. Management's power depends upon how well a strike can be resisted. The power of each is enhanced by careful strike preparations, even though most contracts are resolved time after time without any disruption from strikes.

The actual negotiations are initiated when the employee organization presents the administrator's bargainers with a list of demands. Management may present its own demands or offer counterproposals. Concessions are made by both sides until all issues are resolved or dropped. Management and the union membership then approve the agreement, and a binding contract exists.

If deadlocks occur, the services of a state, federal, or private mediator can be obtained. The mediator tries to conciliate the parties and then mediate their differences.

The contract is a legally enforceable document. Strikes and court actions are two seldom-used means of assuring compliance. More commonly, questions of interpretation are resolved through the grievance and arbitration procedures outlined in the agreement.

POINTS FOR REFLECTION

1. List ten topics that may be included in a contract.
2. Describe the steps union and management go through to prepare for contract negotiations.
3. Describe how union and management may use long-range goals.
4. What are mandatory, voluntary, and illegal collective bargaining issues?
5. Describe the function of mediators in negotiations.

SELECTED READINGS

1. Balke, Walter Morely, Kenneth R. Hammond, and G. Dale Meyer. An alternative approach to labor-management negotiations. *Administrative Science Quarterly* 18:311, 1973.
2. Brookshire, Michael L., and J. Fred Holly. Resolving bargaining impasses through gradual pressure strikes. *Labor Law Journal* 24:662, 1973.
3. Corbett, Laurence P. Mediation arbitration: From the employers standpoint. *Monthly Labor Review* 96:52, 1973.

4. Cullen, Donald E. *Negotiation Labor-Management Contracts* (Bulletin 56). Ithaca, New York: New York State School for Industrial and Labor Relations, 1965.
5. Griffity, M. J. R., Walton M. Hancock, and Fred Munson. Practical ways to contain hospital costs. *Harvard Business Review* 51:131, 1973.
6. Hershfield, David G. Labor relations pressures for equal opportunity. *The Conference Board Record* 10:44, 1973.
7. Lowenberg, Joseph J. Multilateral bargaining: Variation of a theme. *Labor Law Journal* 26:107, 1975.
8. Mironi, Mordechai. The confidentiality of personnel records: A legal and ethical view. *Labor Law Journal* 25:270, 1974.
9. Rausch, Erwin. *Collective Bargaining.* Chicago: Science Research Associates, 1968.
10. Tracy, Lane. The influence on noneconomic factors on negotiators. *Industrial and Labor Relations Review* 27:204, 1974.
11. Vial, Don. Toward a National Health Care System — What's Relevant in the Experience of Negotiated Programs. In James L. Stern and Barbara D. Dennis (Eds.), *Proceedings of the Twenty-Seventh Annual Winter Meeting, Industrial Relations Research Association.* Madison, Wisconsin: Industrial Relations Research Association, 1974. Pp. 17–20.
12. Werther, William B., Jr. A new direction in rethinking fringe benefits. *MSU Business Topics* 22:35, 1974.

8

Administration of the Agreement

Justice delayed is justice denied.
— A legal axiom.

Contract administration follows organizing and negotiations as the third
phase of labor-management relations. It consists of the enforcement and
interpretation of the agreement developed through negotiations. The
contract officially exists at the time both parties sign the document;
but the past practices of management and employees, the constraints
of laws and their interpretations, and the goals of management and union
have all contributed to the development of the presently existing agreement.

The organizing drive and the newly negotiated contract have also
forced administrative adjustments within the organization. Channels
of communication created to counter union activity usually remain open
and are refined with use. Ineffective management policies identified
in the organizing drive are modified, while those left unchanged by the
contract are implicitly accepted.

A multitude of other subjects influences the administration of the
agreement, even though these subjects may or may not be in the written
document. Federal and state laws, management practices, codes of
professional conduct, union standards for craftspeople, safety rules,
and dress codes are commonly excluded but still influential. Many
issues are included in the contract by reference: for example, personnel
policies, letters of explanation, and disciplinary procedures. The contract
wording simply refers to these documents as being accepted by both

parties. Writings included by reference have the same force as clauses stated in the contract [4].

A legally enforceable contract that does not include all relevant rights and responsibilities is frightening. If one cannot look to a single source — or series of sources — to discover the constraints, how is it possible to know what is allowed and prohibited? Providers must assume that everything permitted before the agreement is permitted after the agreement, except for those prohibitions set forth in the contract (in writing or by reference).

People anticipate that collective action within an organization will radically modify the work environment. In practice, changes are evolutionary. The tasks remain essentially the same; subordinates must still follow the orders of superiors. The contract defines the roles of each party more precisely, but this does not cause major changes in day-to-day working relationships. The primary innovation is that employees can effectively protest management decisions that allegedly violate the contract.

The remainder of this chapter explores the causes and resolution of protests under the contract. Complaints are handled through a grievance procedure that allows labor and management to find mutually satisfying settlements. When solutions do not result from this procedure, most agreements call for the use of an outside neutral, an arbitrator, to hear the issues and render a binding decision. If arbitration is not permitted by the contract or if the dispute arises over the negotiation of the agreement, a strike may ensue to obtain resolution. Strikes, alternatives to strikes, and the governmentally imposed notification requirements that are a prerequisite to a strike in a health care facility will be discussed in Chapter 9.

GRIEVANCES

When one party fails to abide by the contract or by accepted past practices, the result is a grievance brought by the other party. Either labor or management may be in the role of wrongdoer. Most grievances, however, are filed against management. The higher number of grievances filed against employers is inherent in the roles played by unions and administrators. It is management's responsibility to make decisions, issue orders, and take action. When an employee does something wrong or violates the contract, the supervisor issues a summary penalty. If the judgment was correct, no complaint occurs. When the supervisory response is perceived as wrong, a grievance is filed. Many of the allegations against management are made because of discipline applied to an employee who acted incorrectly in the first place. Thus, most grievances are against the employer simply because of the active role of management [6].

The role of the union is more passive. Employee representatives do not issue countless orders that could lead to a violation. Once the contract is negotiated, the labor officials take little direct action unless some management decision violates the agreement. When a violation does occur, a grievance results.

GRIEVANCE PROCEDURES

The elements of each grievance procedure are similar, although the details may vary from employer to employer. If a complaint is not resolved in the initial discussion, the grievance is passed on to higher levels of management and union officials. Appeal steps continue until a solution is agreed upon or until all stages of the process have been exhausted.

To illustrate, the following steps are typical of the grievance procedure when a complaint is filed by the union against management, and both sides believe they are right. First, the supervisor takes an action that an employee feels is in violation of contractual rights. The worker talks with the supervisor about the disagreement informally. Failing to get satisfaction, the employee asks the steward to intercede. The steward then attempts to right the wrong through an informal chat with the employee's superior. When the supervisor thinks the original decision was appropriate, the steward makes no progress. At this point the complaint is reduced to writing and filed with the supervisor (within a time period specified by the contract). The supervisor must respond in writing. If the employee wishes to pursue the matter, the steward moves the grievance to the second stage by filing a written complaint with the next level of management. If the original decision is not overturned, and the employee still wishes to pursue it, the issue continues on to a committee.

The committee is composed of union and management representatives. The case is reviewed and either upheld or denied. In the last step of the process the union president and a high-ranking administrator (probably the director of personnel) give the complaint its final joint review. If the decision is still unfavorable to the employee and the union officials think the issue merits further consideration, it is presented to an arbitrator. When the contract does not permit arbitration, the union must either accept the final decision or strike.

In this example, the grievance procedure had five steps:

1. Supervisor and steward and employee
2. Middle manager and steward (with or without employee)
3. Management committee and union grievance committee
4. Top administrator and union president
5. Arbitration

A large hospital with several thousand workers might have a grievance system with six or seven steps. The additional stages include review by successively higher levels of middle management. In a small clinic or nursing home the complaint process might have only three steps. As a rule the larger the organization, the more levels there are to the grievance process, so that the total number of complaints reaching top administrators and union officials is minimized.

TYPES AND CAUSES OF GRIEVANCES

It is important for providers to understand the types and causes of grievances. Different classifications of grievances merit different reactions from managers and union leaders. The final disposition of a complaint is guided by its classification. A reduction in the number of grievances can be achieved only if underlying causes are known. Otherwise the grievance mechanism becomes flooded with repetitive complaints that obscure novel and important ones [15].

Legitimate Grievances

Past practices and the contract constitute a complex web of regulations. Complaints are unavoidable even with the most competent managers and union officials. No matter how knowledgeable and cooperative each side is, reasonable people sometimes disagree over the interpretation or application of rights and responsibilities. When one side violates the understanding between the parties, the resulting grievance is legitimate.

Complaints arise primarily from two sources: ignorance and lack of commitment. The first-level supervisor is evaluated and rewarded on how well the objectives of the institution are met. Labor relations goals are given low priority by the supervisor's superior. The supervisor therefore sees labor relations as being of secondary importance. Thus many first-level managers attempt to give orders without even having read the labor agreement.

The solution is for the top administrator to establish labor relations objectives for each middle manager. These managers then create similar goals for subordinate managers. In addition the personnel or industrial relations department can design training programs that familiarize supervisors with the complexities of the contract.

The problem faced by the union is less severe. Stewards are elected or appointed to their role. They do not obtain that position without first having an interest in labor relations. To the steward, learning and administering the contract is to some degree a privilege. Therefore the steward's motivation for understanding the agreement is usually higher than that of the supervisor who views contract administration as a chore [15].

Imagined Grievances

An imagined grievance occurs when one party incorrectly believes that there has been a violation. Imagined violations are almost always voiced by employees who do not understand their rights. Stewards who are knowledgeable about the contract and its meaning should stop such complaints before they become formal, written grievances. Processing imagined grievances undermines the credibility of the steward and thus of the union. Likewise, if a member of management argues for an imagined grievance, higher level superiors should withdraw the grievance. If this is not done, legitimate complaints may be lumped with imagined grievances and labeled frivolous. Obviously no one benefits from such a situation.

When imagined grievances plague the system, management must initiate a solution. The best response is education. If workers, stewards, and supervisors can be informed of the actual intent behind the language of the legal contract; misunderstandings and resultant imagined grievances can be minimized. Education can occur in training sessions or through supplemental written explanations of the contract. Whatever means is used, the union officials should be consulted. A joint educational effort is more likely to be considered objective by supervisors, stewards, *and* employees.

Political Grievances

Imagined grievances are pursued out of ignorance. Political grievances are fostered for reasons other than the complaint itself. For example, a steward may be reluctant to tell a grievant that the complaint is without merit, since rejecting someone's plea for help may mean a lost vote the next time the steward is up for election. In an extreme case members may desert the union and request a decertification election if they feel they are not getting adequate help.

Managers are guilty of political grievances, too. Those who have appointed someone to a supervisory position are often reluctant to admit that such an appointment might have been an error. A middle manager often feels a need to show subordinate managers that their boss is supportive. Thus a manager may fail to withdraw or concede a grievance to the union because of "how it might look to other members of management." The grievance is evaluated on its political impact and not on its merits [5].

As is the case with imagined grievances, political ones merely overtax the system and diminish the credibility of the instigating party. Unlike imagined grievances, however, politically motivated complaints have no simple solution. There is the possibility that valid grievances may be withheld if too much pressure is brought to bear on the stewards or supervisors by their respective superiors. The only satisfactory resolution of this type of grievance is a cooperative atmosphere between labor and management.

Harassment Grievances

Grievances are sometimes fabricated to harass the other side. Management use of such a technique is infrequent, since the disruption caused detracts from productivity and hurts the institution. Unions may use such practices when, for example, a steward feels management has used unfair tactics to win a grievance case or in the hope that a flood of grievances will cause management to remove an obnoxious supervisor.

The most obvious form of harassment grievances occurs when the union systematically has every steward file petty (or even false) complaints in order to wring a concession from management. Such an institution-wide effort generally occurs only in connection with negotiations. The theory is that the union can demand that every grievance be settled before the contract is signed. As negotiations come down to the hard issues, the union can trade grievances for concessions at the bargaining table.

The only meaningful solution to harassment grievances is to find the underlying causes. Transfers are an answer when the causes center around one or two people. When harassment techniques are used in conjunction with contract negotiations, there is little that can be done. Making a concession encourages such behavior in the future. The standard response is for management to deny all grievances — valid and invalid ones. The union is forced to drop the grievances or request arbitration. If the arbitration clause is worded in a manner that forces both sides to share in the expenses, the harassment grievances are usually not submitted to arbitration.

ARBITRATION

Regardless of the type or cause of a grievance, most contracts permit either party to request arbitration when the complaint is not satisfactorily resolved. The arbitrator can be anyone upon whom both parties agree. Some contracts call for a standing arbitrator who hears every unsettled dispute. This arrangement permits the arbitrator to become familiar with the unique dimensions of a particular union-management relationship. The more common approach, however, is for the parties to contract with an arbitrator to hear a particular case. In this way the arbitrator is under no pressure to "even the score" of wins and losses.

The American Arbitration Association (AAA) and the Federal Mediation and Conciliation Service (FMCS) are the two primary sources of professional arbitrators. The AAA is a nonprofit, nonpartisan organization. Upon request, for a nominal fee, it will provide a list of qualified arbitrators. The association offers other services, such as mediation and expedited arbitration. Expedited arbitration permits a grievance to be resolved within a short time after an impasse is reached [9]. Fact-finding is also available to interested parties. When a deadlock occurs over a grievance (or, more likely, during negotiations), the bargainers may want an objective appraisal of the situation. A neutral fact-finder can perform this function.

The Federal Mediation and Conciliation Service is a government agency primarily involved in mediation of disputes arising out of contract negotiations [2]. It will, however, upon request, make available lists of competent arbitrators.

Whichever source is selected, the payment of the arbitrator's fees and expenses is *not* the responsibility of the FMCS or the AAA. These costs are paid according to the language of the contract. This usually means that management and the union share equally in the costs, but some contracts specify that the loser pays. Both these methods help to prevent political harassment and imagined grievances from reaching arbitration. If the loser pays all, it is a severe financial burden. If one side is in a financially weak position, that side may avoid arbitration simply because of the expense. "Loser-pays-all" clauses can result in justice only for those with healthy treasuries.

Rarely, the contract may state that one side always pays. This arrangement should be avoided, since there is nothing to stop the non-paying side from requesting arbitration on frivolous issues.

Preparation

Arbitration is not automatic. The dissatisfied party must request it. The AAA, the FMCS, or some mutually acceptable person is contacted. When the AAA or FMCS is used, each party gets a list of arbitrators. Those who are not acceptable to either party are struck from the list (usually because of past decisions or because the arbitrator is unknown). The parties choose the arbitrator from the remaining names. The time, date, and place of the arbitration are then set.

Prior to the hearing of the arbitration case, detailed preparations are undertaken by labor and management. These prearbitration activities critically influence the outcome of the case.

Each side must first determine who is to be its representative. If management and union officials present their own cases, the additional cost of legal representation is saved. Whoever does handle the case for either side must undertake specific preparatory actions. The initial grievance must be studied in terms of its cause, its history, and the

* reasons for *both* positions. Relevant parts of the labor contract and other related documents are reviewed.

Witnesses must also be interviewed to assess the nature of the testimony they will give at the hearing. The points each will make should be listed. This assures that favorable testimony is not overlooked during the hearing, since a checklist can be reviewed for each witness before that person is excused. Statements of hostile witnesses must be disproved or at least offset with other information.

The basic principle of debate — prepare your case from the perspective of your opponent — is good advice. It forces one to consider the strengths and weaknesses of both sides and should make it possible to prepare a stronger case.

Documents related to the hearing should be in triplicate — a copy for the arbitrator, a copy for the opponent, and a copy for the presenter. A statement of the major objectives to be achieved during the hearing should be compiled, reviewed, and practiced. This statement clarifies the issues and serves as the basis for the opening remarks. Explaining the case to a confidant who acts as devil's advocate is good practice and may reveal weaknesses in the presentation. Research should include a review of published decisions and the reasoning applied by other arbitrators in similar cases. Past decisions are not binding, but the logic found in other cases may provide an excellent theme. Finally, the attendance of witnesses should be checked a couple of days before the hearing as well as immediately before starting the presentation [10].

Hearing

An arbitration hearing is similar to a courtroom proceeding, although usually much less formal. The arbitrator is sometimes sworn in to add an air of dignity to the process. Rules of evidence normally followed in a court of law are relaxed. Hearsay evidence is often permitted.

The arbitrator usually begins with a few opening remarks to explain the procedure and formality that will be followed. Next the initiating party — the side that requested the hearing — makes an opening statement. This opening statement sets forth the theme, purpose, and conclusion desired by the initiating party. The responding side is given the option of making an opening statement then or reserving it until the respondent presents a case [3]. The next steps are straightforward:

1. Initiating party presents and examines a witness. ·
2. Opposing side cross-examines the witness.
3. Subsequent witnesses for the initiating party are examined and then cross-examined.
4. Responding party presents and examines its first witness.
5. This witness is cross-examined by the initiating party.
6. Subsequent witnesses for the responding party are examined and cross-examined.
7. Initiating party makes a closing statement.
8. Responding party makes a closing statement.

The closing statements, like the opening ones, are merely attempts to point out how the evidence favors one side [10].

Written briefs are submitted to the arbitrator unless both parties agree otherwise. These briefs carefully detail the evidence and show why the case should be decided one way and not another. The arbitrator studies all information — the contract, testimony, similar cases, exhibits, and briefs. A decision is rendered in writing to both sides, usually within a month. (In expedited arbitration [7] written briefs are dispensed with, and the arbitrator may issue a summary judgment shortly after the proceeding or after only a short recess.)

Presentation

Certain techniques observed by experienced arbitrators and labor relations practitioners are helpful in presenting an arbitration case. Although they will not win a weak case, these techniques help in a close decision

First and foremost, it is the arbitrator who must be convinced. Too often the parties start trying to convince their opponent and direct comments at the opponent instead of at the arbitrator. The use of an arbitrator is proof that this technique has failed; comments should be directed to the arbitrator.

Exaggeration is a human weakness. When the presenter of a case resorts to crass exaggeration however, this implies that facts are not enough. It indicates a weak case being argued on the basis of wild, unsupportable claims. Experienced arbitrators will sense that there is little substance behind the emotionalism and conjecture. The best way to demonstrate concern and the desire to win is through careful preparation — not exaggeration, emotionalism, or unsupported opinions.

Witnesses should also be informed of the need for a calm and factual presentation. If a witness lies or exaggerates, this reflects adversely on the case of whoever solicited the person to testify. The witness should be cooperative and courteous with the arbitrator. It is unfortunate, but some arbitrators are influenced by the personality of witnesses and those who present the case.

Cutting Costs

Arbitration is inexpensive compared with court costs. The low cost, speed, and privacy of arbitration make it attractive to labor and management officials. Nevertheless, a simple arbitration case costs several hundred dollars, excluding the value of the time spent by witnesses and those who present the cases. Complex cases easily cost several thousand dollars [12].

Since these expenses are usually borne equally by the parties, cooperation can be mutually advantageous. Dramatic cost reductions can be achieved by following some simple rules.

In advance of the hearing both parties should seek written agreement on as many points as possible and should submit the agreement to the arbitrator. This minimizes a parade of witnesses that only establishes agreed-upon facts. Since the arbitrator's bill is a function of the time devoted to the case, time saved is money saved.

The arbitrator should be asked for a brief written opinion. Some arbitrators are enamored of their own prose. Unless requested to do otherwise, they may write a decision that will prove to be long and therefore costly.

Legal complexities add to arbitration expenses. Whenever possible, union and management officials should present their own cases and avoid the cost of lawyers. The excessive use of legal citations forces the arbitrator to research, study, and evaluate these cases. Again, more time means more expense. A courtroom stenographer employed to transcribe testimony causes delays because written briefs usually are not begun until after the transcript is reviewed. Moreover the cost of the transcript can be a major expense in itself.

Arbitrator's fees are negotiable. If high fees are charged, one of the parties should ask whether the arbitrator would take the case for less. If the answer is no, the parties should consider finding another arbitrator. Many union leaders, managers, and lawyers prefer to use an experienced arbitrator, but obviously a well-known, experienced arbitrator is going to charge more than a less experienced one. In complex cases or cases in which the issues hold significant ramifications for the labor-management relationship, neither side can afford an inexperienced arbitrator. When the dispute is not complex, however, an inexperienced arbitrator may save several hundred dollars of unneeded expenses.

Enforcement

The decision of an arbitrator is enforceable in court. In 1960 the United States Supreme Court ruled in a series of three cases (called the *Trilogy* or *Douglas Doctrine*), that courts were prohibited from overruling an arbitrator when (1) the court thought the issue being arbitrated was frivolous, or (2) the court disagreed with the decision of the arbitrator. As reasoned by Associate Justice Douglas, the parties sought arbitration when they included the arbitration clause in their contract. When the parties contracted with the arbitrator, they sought that arbitrator's judgment. Therefore, once the benefit of an arbitrator's thinking is obtained, the parties should be bound by it.

If it were not for this ruling, the thousands of arbitration cases decided each year would be subject to judicial review. This not only would increase the costs of contract administration but would flood the courts with cases. Arbitration would no longer be the final stage in resolving a grievance but just another intermediate step. Justice for the aggrieved would be further delayed. And, as an old legal axiom states, "Justice delayed is justice denied."

The Douglas doctrine added a new twist to contract language, too. Prior to the trilogy decision, it was common for a contract to list only those items subject to arbitration, all other topics being reserved to management's discretion. After this landmark decision, all items not specifically *excluded* from arbitration were subject to it. If management does not want grievances over subcontracting or wage rates to go to arbitration, for example, the topic has to be excluded in the written agreement. Otherwise the union can file a grievance and demand arbi-

tration if satisfaction is not obtained through the internal grievance
system.

NLRB Deferral

What happens if arbitration has been sought on an unfair labor practice
before the National Labor Relations Board learns of its existence? Should
the employee have filed a charge with the NLRB or pursued the grievance
procedure? What happens if both remedies are pursued simultaneously?
Which decision dominates?

The NLRB has established precedents in such situations. If the Board
does not learn of the unfair labor practice charge until after the issue has
been arbitrated, the NLRB will review the arbitrator's decision. The
NLRB allows the arbitrator's decision to stand if the decision is binding
on both labor and management, if the proceedings were fair, and if the
arbitrator's decision was not repugnant to the purposes of the labor laws.
When any of these elements are missing, the NLRB will initiate its own
investigation. This procedure is sometimes called the *Spielberg Manufacturing Doctrine* after one of the parties in the case in which the board
established this approach [8].

Under the *Collyer Insulated Wire* case the Board knew of an unfair
labor practice allegation before it was arbitrated. In that case, the NLRB
retained jurisdiction until after the arbitration decision. Again the Board
applied the same standards: the decision had to be binding, fair, and not
repugnant to the labor laws [11].

When an individual believes an unfair labor practice has occurred, he
should check first with the local office of the National Labor Relations
Board. If for some reason this cannot be done within the time limit required to file a grievance, the employee should initiate a grievance charge
and then check with the NLRB as soon as possible [13]. This allows the
NLRB jurisdiction over the case if it chooses to have it.

SUMMARY

Contract administration is the third phase of labor-management relations.
Although organizing and negotiations establish many rules, most past
management practices remain unchanged. The contract merely modifies
some practices. The process is evolutionary, not revolutionary.

Typically the central concern of contract administration is resolving disputes that arise from the interpretation of the agreement. It is rare for such problems to be solved by a strike. In almost every case the complainant resorts to the grievance procedure.

The grievance process is a series of steps through which complaints are aired and usually satisfied. When it fails, arbitration is the final stage. A neutral hears the issues and renders an enforceable decision.

A strike is an alternative only when the contract lacks a no-strike clause. Even then, lengthy notification procedures must be adhered to if the strike is to be considered a protected activity. More commonly, strikes happen as a result of a breakdown in contract negotiations. Since strikes are an important tool and most providers are unaware of the implications surrounding them, the next chapter will explore the topic of strikes and notification requirements.

POINTS FOR REFLECTION

1. What are the three phases of health care labor relations?
2. Describe the grievance procedure and its purposes.
3. What are the types of grievances?
4. Describe the process of arbitration over grievances.
5. How is jurisdiction over unfair labor practices determined between an arbitrator and the NLRB?

SELECTED READINGS

1. Coulson, Robert. The emerging role of title VII arbitration. *Labor Law Journal* 26:263, 1975.
2. Corbett, Laurence P. Mediation/arbitration: From the employer's standpoint. *Monthly Labor Review* 96:52, 1973.
3. Glasser, Joseph. An analysis of the arbitration procedure. *Personnel Journal* 52:976, 1973.
4. Goldfinger, Nat. Labor-Management Relations in an Increasingly Difficult Economic Environment (Presidential Address to the Twenty-Seventh Annual Winter Meeting of the Industrial Relations Research Association). In James L. Stern and Barbara D. Dennis (Eds.), *Proceedings of the Twenty-Seventh Annual Winter Meeting*. Madison, Wisconsin: Industrial Relations Research Association, 1974.
5. Jennings, Ken. Foremen's views of their involvement with other

management officials in the grievance process. *Labor Law Journal* 25:305, 1974.
6. Jennings, Ken. Foremen's views of their involvement with the union steward in the grievance process. *Labor Law Journal* 25:540, 1974.
7. Kane, Steven E. Current developments in expedited arbitration. *Labor Law Journal* 24:282, 1973.
8. Nash, Peter G. Board referral to arbitration and Alexander v. Denver: Some preliminary observations. *Labor Law Journal* 25:259, 1974.
9. American Arbitration Association. *Expedited Labor Arbitration Rules of the American Arbitration Association.* New York (no date).
10. American Arbitration Association. *Labor Arbitration: Procedures and Techniques.* New York (no date).
11. Pye, Rosemary. Collyer's effect on the individual charging party. *Labor Law Journal* 25:561, 1974.
12. Rubenstein, Benjamin. Some thoughts about arbitration costs. *Labor Law Journal* 24:362, 1973.
13. Siber, Bonnie L. The Gardner-Denver decision: Does it put arbitration in a bind? *Labor Law Journal* 25:708, 1974.
14. Spelfogel, Evan J. Wildcat strikes and minority concerted activity: Discipline, damage suits and injunctions. *Labor Law Journal* 24:592, 1973.
15. Werther, William B., Jr. Reducing grievances through effective contract administration. *Labor Law Journal* 25:211, 1974.

9

Strikes, Lockouts, and Notification

All power is a trust.
— Benjamin Disraeli

The strike is a powerful and last-ditch effort used when contract negotiations fail. In negotiations the employee organization must either accept management's offer or strike. Even so, strikes are rare. During the last twenty-five years less than 1 percent of the time available for work in the United States has been lost because of strikes [18]. Almost all contract negotiations are concluded peacefully, as are nearly all grievances in labor-management agreements. In fact strikes are so uncommon that it is newsworthy when one does occur. For every strike reported by the media, hundreds of disputes are amicably settled.

Strikes do occur, but in most industries the concerted action is an inconvenience that soon passes. Repercussions for the public, the employer, and the workers are seldom catastrophic. In the health care industry, however, the implications for the public can be disastrous even during short strikes.

Recognition of this unique aspect of the health care industry led Congress to impose special notification requirements upon providers. Lengthy and detailed procedures must be followed before either a strike or a lockout is legally permissible. Failure to comply with these requirements can result in strikers' losing the protection of the NLRB. On the other hand if management fails to abide by notification rules, the employer can be forced to fire replacements and pay strikers back wages. Thus the power exercised by both union and management is constrained by law for the benefit of the public [2].

This chapter discusses notification requirements and the types of strikes typically encountered in health care facilities. Alternatives to strikes — alternatives that resolve disputes without "open warfare" — will be presented to offer providers meaningful options.

NOTIFICATION REQUIREMENTS

The 1974 health care amendments to the Labor Management Relations Act set forth legally mandated notification procedures. The purpose of these regulations is to minimize strike-caused disruptions to the delivery of health care. The time limitations vary depending upon whether an existing contract is to be modified (renegotiated) or an initial contract is to be negotiated. Each is examined separately.

Termination or Modification

When an existing contract is to be terminated or modified, the party (labor or management) that intends to terminate or modify it must serve the other party a written notice ninety days in advance of the end of the contract or, when no expiration date exists, from the proposed date of the termination or modification.

Sixty days before the termination or modification the Federal Mediation and Conciliation Service (FMCS) and the appropriate state or territorial agency must be notified, if the parties have not reached an agreement. The FMCS is required by law to communicate with the parties promptly in an attempt to effect an agreement.

During the ninety-day period the employer is not permitted to lock out the employees and the workers are not permitted to strike. If this ninety-day ban is violated, the wrongdoer is guilty of an unfair labor practice. The law requires that the existing contract remain in force during this period unless a mutually satisfactory modification is reached.

A strike, if it does occur, cannot commence until after the ninety-day period has passed. Ten days before the actual strike the employee organization must notify the employer and the FMCS in writing that a strike will begin on a certain date at a specific time. Failure to give the ten-day notice is an unfair labor practice according to section 8(g). This ULP applies only to the health care industry. The notice may be extended by a mutual, written agreement between labor and management.

In summary, the party wishing to change or terminate a labor agreement must notify the other party ninety days before the date of modification or termination. Sixty days before the changes are to occur the FMCS and state or territorial agencies must be notified if no agreement has been reached. Ten days before a strike, a notice must be served on the other party and the FMCS. Under no circumstances may a strike occur during the ninety-day period or without the separate ten-day notice.

Initial Contracts

Notification requirements are shortened when an initial labor agreement is in the process of negotiation. Thirty days before the planned termination of services by either side, the initiating party must notify the FMCS, the appropriate state or territorial mediation agency, and the other party. Once again the FMCS will attempt to resolve the dispute. If the disagreement persists, the parties will be free to engage in strikes and lockouts after the thirty days have expired. As is the case with the renegotiation of contracts, the party planning to withdraw its services must provide a ten-day written notice to the other side and the FMCS.

Factfinding

The health care amendments allow the director of the FMCS to establish an impartial board of inquiry. The purpose of the board is to investigate the issues surrounding the dispute and provide a written report to the parties within fifteen days. The report presents the board's findings of fact and its recommendations for resolving the dispute. These results are not binding on labor and management; each is free to accept or reject the solutions suggested in the report. For fifteen days following the report, however, strikes and lockouts are not permitted. This prohibition supersedes the ten-day notification of an intent to strike; strikes and lockouts are banned for fifteen days even if a ten-day notification has been submitted. Factfinding boards are to be created whenever a strike or threatened strike would substantially impair the delivery of health care in a given area.

Fifteen days following the board's report or ten days after a notification of intent to strike (whichever is later), the union is free to resort to an *economic strike* in order to resolve their differences. The notification procedures assure the involvement of the FMCS and may even lead to the establishment of a board of inquiry, which will delay a strike. Nothing in the law, however, guarantees that strikes will not eventually occur in any labor-management relationship.

Either party that fails to follow notification procedures in a strike will be charged with committing an unfair labor practice. This failure can cause an otherwise legal strike to be considered in violation of the labor laws — specifically, an 8(g)ULP.

TYPES OF STRIKES

Section 7 of the National Labor Relations Act permits employees to join together for their own mutual aid and protection. Normally this means that they are free to engage in what is called an *economic strike,* if no other laws are violated. During economic strikes the law affords the strikers certain protection. However, if a strike results from (or is prolonged by) an unfair labor practice *by a union,* the strikers have no rights under the law. Conversely, if a strike is called because of an unfair labor practice *by management,* the workers are granted the highest form of protection under the law. Thus the differences between *economic* and *unfair labor practice* strikes are important to all providers.

Economic Strikes

An economic strike is caused by the concerted efforts of employees to withdraw their services in order to pursue their mutual aid or protection legally. This means that the object of the strike must be legal. When workers engage in concerted action in order to force an employer to undertake an illegal act, this is not an economic strike. For example, nationwide political strikes — common in other countries — are not considered economic strikes.

Besides having a legal end, the strike must use legal means. A strike enacted without the notification process previously described, irrespective of the objective, would not be considered an economic strike.

When an economic strike commences, the employer is free to replace the strikers with new workers and is under no obligation to remove the replacements in favor of the striking employees at the conclusion of the strike. If, when openings occur, management refuses to rehire the strikers because of their strike actions, however, the employer is guilty of an unfair labor practice. Management can replace economic strikers but may not discriminate against them in the future. If replacements have not been hired, management must reinstate strikers who reapply for work after the strike.

Some sympathy strikes are considered to be the same as economic strikes. When organized workers strike in sympathy with another union, the result is an economic strike. Such would be the case if LPN's struck in sympathy with nurses, for example. Here again, acceptable means and ends must be employed by the strikers. Otherwise the strike may be considered an unfair labor practice strike.

Unfair Labor Practice Strikes

There are two types of unfair labor practice strikes: those caused or prolonged by a union's unfair labor practice and those caused or prolonged by an employer's unfair labor practice.

An unfair labor practice strike caused by a union leaves strikers outside the protection of the NLRB. If the employees' actions provide the employer with grounds for discharge, the workers may be fired. Discharge is not automatic; management may choose either to exercise or to waive this right. An example of grounds for discharge is a sit-down strike in which strikers refuse to leave an employer's property. Another example is a strike causing employees to commit a violation that is grounds for termination (such as failure to report to work). Should health care workers strike and fail to provide the required ten-day prior notice, they are involved in an unfair labor practice strike. Under any of these circumstances administrators not only may hire replacements, but they are free to reject the application of the strikers after the strike is ended.

Unfair labor practice strikes caused by management have an opposite effect on workers. If employees initiate an economic strike, for example, and during the strike the employer commits a ULP, the strike becomes an unfair labor practice strike. This leads to the highest level of NLRB protection. Once it is proved that the strike involves unfair labor practice by management, the employer will be required to rehire every striker. This may even lead to the dismissal of replacements to make room for reinstated strikers. Moreover it is common for the NLRB to grant strikers back wages for those working hours missed because of the ULP strike. Common examples of employer unfair labor practices during strikes include management's refusal to bargain in good faith or locking out the members during the ninety-day period before the contract terminates. A strike may be initiated by the union in response to a management unfair labor practice; it is not necessary that the action start out as an economic strike.

INJUNCTIONS AGAINST STRIKES

When strikes violate court decrees, labor laws, or other laws, the rights of the innocent party may be legally enforced. The procedures used to control strikes depend on the labor contract and federal statutes. An examination of improper strikes and their remedies further underscores the fact that the right to strike is limited.

The principle goal, when an illegal strike occurs, is to stop it. The legal device that can do this is called a *temporary restraining order*. This is a judicial decree prohibiting a strike under the threat of a contempt of court charge should the strike continue. In time a hearing is held on the temporary restraining order to determine whether it should be replaced by a permanent injunction or simply dropped.

Prior to 1932, and the passage of the Norris-LaGuardia (Anti-Injunction) Act, federal courts were liberal in granting injunctions to employers. This severely limited the effectiveness of the strike weapon. Once the Norris-LaGuardia Act became law, it became increasingly difficult for employers to secure an injunction in a labor dispute.

When an unfair labor practice strike occurs, the NLRB can request – upon showing cause – an injunction from a federal district court. It is virtually impossible for a union or employer to secure such an injunction for unfair labor practice strikes.

An injunction can be obtained when a strike arises over issues that are the proper subject of the grievance procedure or arbitration. This assumes that the strike is also a breach or violation of the contract [16]. The United States Supreme Court has spelled out the steps necessary to obtain an injunction under these circumstances. In a 1970 case, *Boys Markets, Inc. v. Retail Clerks*, it was decided that the following conditions must exist before an injunction can be issued by a federal court.

1. There is a contractual obligation to arbitrate the issue.
2. The employer will be required to arbitrate the dispute as a condition of securing the injunction.
3. There has been a violation of the no-strike provisions of the labor agreement.
4. The employer will suffer more if the injunction is denied than the union will if the injunction is granted.
5. The violations of the contract have resulted in irreparable damage to the employer.

Although injunctions are still used, they are not common. In health care labor relations they are issued typically when one of the parties violates the ninety-day or ten-day notification period.

ALTERNATIVES TO STRIKES

Strikes are rapidly becoming an anachronism [12]. In a highly specialized society mutual interdependence between institutions is an undeniable reality. The disruption of a strike in a major institution is felt throughout the community. The repercussions impair the functioning of other institutions, the employer, and the strikers themselves. The strike-impaired organization faces a decline in revenue which leaves it less able to meet the demands of society and the strikers. The strikers' financial situation deteriorates. At the conclusion of the strike the winner often has a Pyrrhic victory; the gain is small compared with the costs of obtaining the gain [8].

The hardships caused by strikes would be acceptable in a free society if they were limited to the direct participants. Workers and their employer could be left to decide how much suffering they were willing to accept. However, strikes affect the public, and nowhere is this more obvious than in the health care field.

If strikes begin to seriously disrupt the delivery of health care across a wide number of communities, political action in inevitable. Whenever one group in society is abused by another, legislation intervenes to redress the imbalance of power. The labor laws, civil rights laws, age discrimination legislation, and health and safety enactments are examples of this. The American legislative system is a delicate balance of advocacies between those with power and those without it. If the relatively powerless public is seriously jeopardized by strikes in the health care field, strikes will be outlawed. Alternatives to strikes will be imposed. The object of these alternatives will be to reduce strikes; their appeal to providers will be of only secondary consideration. Unrestrained use of strikes in the health field will lead to withdrawal of the privilege.

It is incumbent upon providers, therefore, to minimize strikes, not only because of the harm caused the providers themselves by work stoppages but because of the potential loss of freedom to resolve labor-management disputes through strikes. Although there is no one alternative to strikes that is universally applicable to all health care facilities, each alternative has its advantages [21].

Binding Arbitration

Binding arbitration is the least desirable of the available alternatives. A contract dispute submitted to an arbitrator may result in a binding decree that displeases *both* labor and management. Too often an arbitrator attempts to "split the difference" between the parties in a misguided effort to be fair. This may mean that desired management prerogatives are lost as well as a meaningful package of wages and benefits for union members. Furthermore, for employers dealing with multiple unions or unions dealing with multiple employers, decrees by different arbitrators may lead to widely varying treatment, causing resentment and morale problems among rank-and-file employees [14].

If binding arbitration is to be pursued in contract disputes, it is in the interest of the parties to specify issues the arbitrator is permitted to decide. Obviously if agreement can be reached on critical issues that are not subject to arbitration without an arbitrator, the parties can probably resolve most of the remaining issues without an arbitrator [6].

Binding arbitration does have some advantages. If nothing else, it results in a resolution of negotiation deadlocks without the disruption of a strike. Since both parties know the arbitrator's decision may be less than optimal, it encourages compromises and meaningful negotiations as the deadline for submission to arbitration nears [15]. Topics already agreed upon are not submitted to an arbitrator. Therefore the parties may find a compromise more appealing than the possibility of an even less favorable decision by an arbitrator [9].

Final Offer

A variant of simple binding arbitration is the final offer approach. Here union and management officials reach agreement on as many items as possible. Deadlocked issues are then submitted to an arbitrator. The arbitrator is allowed to pick only the most reasonable package of proposals, selecting either management's or the union's last offer [22]. The arbitrator is not allowed to substitute a third alternative.

Such arbitration forces parties to close the gap between them. If the union is asking for an absurdly high settlement and management's offer is ridiculously low, each side knows it must reach a more reasonable position. In adjusting their positions, the two sides may reach a compromise that leads to settlement without arbitration. Even if arbitration does occur, the differences may be narrowed sufficiently to allow the final decision to be satisfying for both management and the union members [17].

In final offer arbitration there is an incentive to close the gap between the relative positions. In binding arbitration, on the other hand, there is an advantage to staying far apart. If management's offer is reasonable and the union's is unreasonable, binding arbitration may cause the difference to be split. Thus the winner becomes the side that compromised the least. In final offer arbitration the winning side is the one that has made the most reasonable offer.

Med-arb

Med-arb is an abbreviation for *mediation-arbitration*. Under this technique, the arbitrator joins the parties well before they are to submit their disagreements to arbitration. During the prearbitration phase the arbitrator acts as mediator and attempts to keep the parties talking. Hard feelings and threats to walk out of meetings are soothed in order to keep negotiations going. Compromises are suggested and priorities assessed. If negotiations do not conclude by some predetermined date, or if the parties feel they have reached a deadlock, the mediator then assumes the role of arbitrator and produces a decision based on inside information to which an arbitrator would not, under normal circumstances, have been privy [4].

This approach has the advantage of making the arbitrator intimately familiar with the wishes of both sides and the problems inherent in the situation. Therefore a more realistic solution should be forthcoming. Unfortunately this method is expensive, although less costly than a strike [11]. Also, if the parties intentionally misstate their positions, the decree could be unfair. For example, if in a private conference the union tells the mediator-arbitrator that it must have a minimum of 12 percent, and management claims that 8 percent is its maximum, the arbitrator may compromise at 10 percent. Realizing this possible outcome, the parties have an incentive to understate or overstate their positions. This again leads to the possibility of the more unrealistic position being rewarded. Nothing requires the arbitrator to split the difference, however. If, in the above example, the arbitrator believed that 9 percent was fair for both sides, the final decision would be 9 percent. When the major problems submitted for arbitration center around nonmonetary items such as contract language or working conditions, med-arb leads to a more realistic decision than any other alternative involving outsiders [13].

Nonstoppage Strikes

Many management and union officials cringe at the thought of bringing in someone to render a decision on the terms of a contract. The loss of power is in itself threatening. More significantly there is the real possibility that the parties will be stuck with a decision that is unacceptable and binding.

One way to avoid a strike as well as the risk of an outsider's decision is to declare a *nonstoppage strike*. When this method is used, a strike commences as soon as the contract expires or negotiations reach a deadlock. The difference is that the strike is on paper; the performance of the organization is unaffected, and workers continue to work. However, they are all paid the minimum wage, not their regular wage or salary. This puts pressure on the union to come to an agreement with management. At the same time the organization is assessed a penalty — for example, 50 percent of all revenue earned during the strike. The organization's penalty and the workers' regular pay (less the minimum wage) are turned over to a trustee. To add pressure for a settlement, the trustee can be directed to turn the monies over to some designated charity as an irrevocable gift at the end of thirty days if no agreement is reached.

The amount of the penalties and their final disposition is crucial. Labor and management should negotiate these points separately from contract negotiations. The advantage to nonstoppage strikes is that labor and management decide everything between themselves [20]. Their penalties serve to force a settlement without disruption to the delivery of health care or potentially unsatisfactory decisions by arbitrators.

Experimental Negotiations Agreement

Realizing that strikes were harming employees, member companies, and the American economy, the steel industry and its unions tried a novel technique that was labeled an experimental negotiations agreement (ENA). Although developed in the steel industry, it could prove beneficial to the health care industry.

Both sides agree that at the expiration of the contract there will be no strike or lockout. In return for labor's pledge not to strike, management agrees to give an automatic wage increase upon the termination of the contract. This raise is minimal, and both parties realize it is not the final offer. The provisions of the old contract — work rules, fringe benefits, and so forth — remain in force. Starting with the first pay date following the expiration, the workers are given a marginal increase of 3 or 4 percent. Labor and management continue to negotiate free of outside influence. When an accord is obtained, the final increase is granted retroactively, so there is no penalty for the workers and no advantage for management to delaying the settlement [1]. There are no outsiders; there are no expenses related to arbitration; there is no disruption in service; and there are no hard feelings among clients, suppliers, and the public. Simply put, no one loses. The result in the steel industry is that there will be no nationwide strikes for the remainder of the 1970's.

Combinations

There is nothing to prevent any combination of these various strike alternatives. Union and management officials could agree to use final offer arbitration for wage issues and med-arb for all other items not resolved. The ENA technique could be combined with a modified nonstoppage strike to assure no disruptions but still keep the pressure on both sides for a prompt solution.

Although traditional strikes do lead to a resolution of disputes, they are an antiquated concept that is costly to labor, management, and the public. Sometimes, as happened in the steel industry, the cost of strikes is more than the parties wish to bear. In other cases strikes are outlawed because the costs to society are too high — as with most essential government services. No one can deny that health care is essential. If strikes become increasingly common, the freedom of providers will be restricted in favor of the public welfare. There are viable alternatives already in existence that should be considered by providers. Otherwise, it is possible, even probable, that the option to strike that is now enjoyed by providers will be greatly restricted by government fiat [12].

SUMMARY

Strikes are a potent weapon. Unfortunately they create numerous problems for employers, strikers, and the public. Since the disruption of health care is one obvious and serious implication, Congress established stringent notification procedures to minimize the repercussions and eliminate the use of surprise strikes.

The notification requirements demand that, when a collective agreement already exists, the initiating party must notify the other side at least ninety days before the proposed contract changes are to take effect. When an initial contract is being negotiated, the notification must be given at least thirty days prior to the implementation of the changes in the contract. In addition state and federal mediation services must be notified. Ten days before a strike is to commence, the time and date of the action must be communicated to the employer and the FMCS. It is hoped that these advance warnings will cause the parties to undertake negotiations soon enough to avoid a strike. Even when a strike cannot be avoided, there is sufficient time for the health care facility to minimize the disruption caused by the employees' concerted action.

Since strikes in the health care field carry such awesome implications for the public, their uncontrolled use will very likely lead to restrictive legislation. Even if strikes occur seldom, there are strong economic motivations to consider alternatives.

The possible number of substitutes for strikes is limited only by the imagination of providers. Arbitration in any of several forms can be relied upon to resolve impasses. Other techniques include nonstoppage strikes or agreements to extend the present contract until a new one is reached. Modifications and combinations of these alternatives are also possible. The important point is for providers to realize that traditional strikes are but one of many possible means to overcome deadlocks.

POINTS FOR REFLECTION

1. What are the strike notification requirements for the health care industry?
2. Why are the requirements so much more detailed than in other industries?
3. What types of strikes may occur?
4. How are strike rules and regulations enforced?
5. What alternatives can be used instead of strikes?
6. Why must alternatives be considered?

SELECTED READINGS

1. Abel, I. W. Basic steel's experimental negotiating agreement. *Monthly Labor Review* 96:39, 1973.
2. Bennett, George. The elusive public interest in labor disputes. *Labor Law Journal* 25:673, 1974.
3. Cole, David L. The search for industrial peace. *Monthly Labor Review* 96:37, 1973.
4. Corbett, Laurence P. Mediation/arbitration from the employer's standpoint. *Monthly Labor Review* 96:52, 1973.
5. Dunlap, Karen. Mediation-arbitration: Reaction from rank and file *Monthly Labor Review* 96:65, 1973.
6. Flemming, Robbin W. Interest arbitration revisited. *Michigan Business Review* 25:1, 1973.
7. Grunsky, Robert R. Replacing economic weapons with reason. *Monthly Labor Review* 96:53, 1973.
8. Hammermesh, Daniel S. Who "wins" in wage bargaining? *Industrial and Labor Relations Review* 26:1146, 1973.
9. Haughton, Ronald W. Some successful uses of "interest" arbitration. *Monthly Labor Review* 96:60, 1973.
10. Hodgson, James D. Stretching out the duration of labor contracts. *Monthly Labor Review* 96:54, 1973.
11. Kagel, Sam. Combining mediation and arbitration. *Monthly Labor Review* 96:62, 1973.

12. Kheel, Theodore W.   Is the strike outmoded? *Monthly Labor Review* 96:35, 1973.
13. Rollard, Harry.   Mediation-arbitration: A trade union view. *Monthly Labor Review* 96:63, 1973.
14. Seitz, Peter.   Mandatory contract arbitration: A viable process or not, it works (sometimes). *Industrial and Labor Relations Review* 26:1146, 1973.
15. Simkin, William W.   Limitations of arms-length or adversary arbitra tion. *Monthly Labor Review* 96:56, 1973.
16. Spelfogel, Evan J.   Wildcat strikes and minority concerted activity: Discipline, damage suits and injunctions. *Labor Law Journal* 24:592, 1973.
17. Stern, James L.   Final-offer arbitration — Initial experience in Wisconsin. *Monthly Labor Review* 97:39, 1974.
18. United States Department of Labor.   Work stoppages, 1946 to date. *Monthly Labor Review* 98:109, 1975.
19. Usery, William J., Jr.   A more activist approach by mediators. *Monthly Labor Review* 96:59, 1973.
20. Werther, William B., Jr.   Can strikes be made to work for management, labor, and the public? *Industrial Management* 17(9):1, 1975.
21. Winpisinger, William W.   There is no alternative to the right to strike. *Monthly Labor Review* 96:59, 1973.
22. Witney, Fred.   Final-offer arbitration: The Indianapolis experience. *Monthly Labor Review* 96:20, 1973.

10

Cooperation

The longest journey begins with the first step.
  — Ancient Chinese Proverb

Labor-management relations are often viewed as a zero-sum relationship. That is, one side wins only at the expense of the other. Employees obtain higher wages by forcing the employer to accept smaller profits or net revenues; management prerogatives are secured at the expense of less freedom for the union. This mentality leads to a negative arrangement; each side loses and neither gains. Strikes are a prime example. The ideal situation is for administrators, union officials, and rank-and-file members to make sure everyone benefits. This kind of relationship is more than just a different perspective. It offers tangible rewards for all providers.

Most labor-management relationships focus on how to slice "the pie of available benefits." Each side is so concerned about getting a larger slice that the size of the pie is overlooked. Too much effort is expended in a zero-sum arrangement in which benefits accrue only at a cost to the other party. Efforts aimed at increasing surplus revenues would create more benefits for workers and the organization, regardless of the proportions of each slice. This is not to suggest that administrators or union officials should allow the other to dictate contract or grievance settlements. However, in evaluating the employment relationship, it becomes obvious that the largest gains for the members, union, *and* the organization are down the road of cooperation.

BACKGROUND OBSTACLES TO COOPERATION

Unfortunately mistrust and resentment between labor and management exist even before unionization. When unionization occurs, administrators see it as a threat to their ability to manage and a rejection of their past efforts to aid workers. They add to this conventional wisdom a stereotyped view of union officials and demands. Likewise, union leaders see administrative reactions as a rejection of union aspirations.

Once the organizing drive begins, management resists. Both subtle and direct remarks by administrators discourage employees from joining the union. If labor leaders have less formal education and less status than managers, these differences are exploited in management's attempts to relegate labor leaders to a subservient role. Attempts by employee leaders to carve out an area of authority within the institution are seen by administrators as an attack on management's prerogatives. Rather quickly it becomes impossible to discern causes from effects as each side acts and reacts.

People do tire of these games, and at some point someone attempts a reconciliation. No matter who initiates it, the other side is suspicious. After months or years of intolerance and open resentment, cooperative gestures are seen as deceptions. The initiator, once rebuffed, resorts to previous approaches. This reinforces the other side's suspicion that the original move was merely a trick. Each of these attitudes creates confusion and mistrust.

Labor laws and the need to deal with each other act as restraints upon further escalation of the conflict. If the underlying economics become too distorted, the alternatives are renewed cooperation or dissolution through bankruptcy. There are countless cases in which a union and management began to cooperate when it appeared that the survival of the relationship was threatened. When cooperation is attempted by *both* sides, the reaction of each is often, "Why didn't we do this before?"

Admittedly, cooperation will not solve all labor-management problems nor will it cure problems of ineffective management. In many ways, however, both parties can benefit by assisting each other.

The barriers to cooperative effort are many. This chapter describes some of the obstacles that each side is capable of putting in the way of the other. If labor leaders and administrators can recognize and avoid creating these obstacles, the escalation of mistrust and resentment will stop. It may then become possible to implement joint projects that benefit all providers, improve the delivery of health care, and win public support.

PRECAUTIONS FOR MANAGEMENT

Managers who seek the benefits of cooperation often infringe certain labor laws in their zest to change the labor-management atmosphere. Regardless of good intentions, it is still an unfair labor practice for management to dominate a labor organization through financial or nonfinancial means. One manager, in an attempt to express a new-found spirit of cooperation, decided to give the organization's vending machines to the union. The machines had depreciated to their residual scrap value and were essentially valueless. Furthermore management saw no need to provide a food-vending service to employees if the union would do so. The union agreed, and management signed the machines over to the employee organization. A disgruntled union member complained to the NLRB, and management ended by capitulating to an 8(a)(2) charge of domination because the act of giving the machines to the union was, technically, a labor law violation. Had management *not* immediately conceded a technical violation of the labor laws, a considerable amount of money might have been spent on legal fees to fight the case — to fight to be cooperative with the union. Any cooperative action by management must be viewed against the backdrop of the labor laws.

Three concerns that *every* supervisor, *every* middle-level manager, and *every* top administrator should be made aware of in attempting to cooperate with the union are the following:

1. Survival needs of the union.
2. Political needs of the union.
3. Precedent-setting practices.

Survival Needs

Every organization — hospitals, nursing homes, and especially unions — has survival needs. These needs can be categorized into those of the organization, of the leaders, and of the members.

Leaders and members realize that the union provides them with many satisfactions. To members it is an answer to certain needs for security and belonging. It gives them a common identity. To the leader the union is a source of status, pride, and recognition. Attempts by management to undermine the union become a threat to the needs of leaders and members. Thus, when management actions lead to layoffs, moving of the facility, or rejection of the union's request for union shop or some other form of security, union reaction is strong. Why would workers endure a strike for a union security clause? For much the same reason that managers sometimes work ninety hours a week during a strike: dedication to their organization. The organization is a major source of satisfaction for workers and managers alike. When the organization is threatened, its members respond. Managers should consider decisions in terms of their impact on the employee organization.

The role of the union leaders is another area management tends to overlook. When a change is to be implemented, administrators sometimes fail to check with the appropriate union officials. The matter may be nothing more complex than moving a machine to a new location. But if the union is not consulted, and if rank-and-file members then check with the steward, union officials and members may well resent having been left out. To assert leadership (and to obtain the recognition the steward thinks should be forthcoming), the steward may file a grievance over a contractual technicality. (For example, if the supervisor moves the machine, the grievance may state that the work should have been done by a union member in the maintainance department.) Management, not realizing that the action unintentionally undermined the steward's position, cannot understand why the union is so uncooperative. Likewise, the steward cannot understand why the supervisor is so indifferent to the steward's leadership role.

This does not mean that management must seek the steward's approval for every action. If the object is cooperation, however, it is not furthered by unilateral decisions. Management should reinforce the union official's position by at least informing appropriate union leaders first of planned changes. This allows the steward (or other union officials) to maintain credibility as a leader and makes it less likely that minor actions will be perceived as a threat.

The third survival need is that of the members. This is the one need most managers realize quickly. They know that if a disciplinary action is taken against a rank-and-file member, the union will respond. The nature of that response can be influenced in several ways. First, any decision that is detrimental to the members should be substantiated with witnesses or documentation. Second, if the supervisor explains the reason for the action to the appropriate union leader before implementing it, the action will be less threatening to the union and other members. Third, if good documentation always precedes management actions, the union official is less likely to file a complaint to see if management's decision is justified. The steward or other union leader will sense rather quickly that management can prove its case or that it would not take such actions.

Management at all levels must consider the survival needs of the union organization, its leaders, and its members *before* taking action. Failure to do so breeds mistrust between the union and management.

Political Needs

The union is a political organization. Its leaders are elected officials who retain their position (i.e., survive) by winning the support of their constituents. This can lead to a variety of situations that an administrator would label as illogical at first glance. Grievances are filed when it is obvious that management is right, or the union strikes for a minor point in contract negotiations. Underlying political considerations may be the true cause of such acts. Possibly the union leaders need to show the rank and file that they support every member. They may need to use power to assure others they are still in control. Even more simply, union leaders may be merely reflecting the wishes of their constituents.

The standard management response to "irrational" union moves is too often paranoia: "The union is trying to create trouble again." It is much more probable that the political realities of the union are being observed. Generally unions do not harass management intentionally except in response to a management action that they consider ill advised.

Precedents

For political and survival reasons, the union must represent its members. Much like a good defense attorney, the union tries to win for its clients.

Union leaders will sometimes admit that they knew a member was wrong but felt that each member deserves the best defense possible. Nowhere is there more true than in a discharge case. When a worker is discharged, the members watch the union's response. The credibility of the leaders is at stake. If the union appears indifferent to the plight of the discharged worker, the rank and file may lose faith in the union or at least in its leaders. The union leaders must put on a defense.

What hurts management in such situations is not the fact that the union goes through the motions; instead it is management's past practices. If the violation for which the employee has been discharged led only to a written warning in a previous case involving another employee, the union can argue that the employer waived the right to fire workers for that offense. Even if top administrators do not accept that argument, most arbitrators are impressed by it. It is usually judged to be unfair to fire one worker for a given offense when others have received lesser penalties for similar infractions.

It is imperative that management develop and follow a uniform personnel policy in dealing with workers. When exceptions are made — and they should be rare — it must be emphasized to the union leaders and workers that the case is exceptional and not a waiver of management's prerogatives.

Cooperation is much more likely to succeed if the industrial relations environment is one of fair and consistent treatment. When discipline and other actions by employers appear to be capricious, the reaction of union members is one of hostility and caution, not cooperation.

PRECAUTIONS FOR THE UNION

In attempting to be cooperative with management, some union leaders lose their positions. If the rank and file think there is a sweetheart arrangement between top union and administrative people, the leader will be replaced with a "firebrand" [7]. It does not matter what the actual relationship is. If it *appears* too cozy, the rank and file will feel betrayed. Thus a constant concern of union leaders is that they must pursue and *appear* to be pursuing the employees' objectives.

Other than the potential problems for leaders, the union has little to lose by cooperation. Success for the employer carries with it the implied agreement that the workers will share in the benefits. Any management sensitive to the political needs of unions will grant the union leader much of the credit for improvements. If cooperation is used to further the goals of the facility and not the employees, the resulting union harassment will destroy the basis for cooperation. If management violates the contract, even with the tacit approval of the union, in order to obtain better performance, the union can always file a grievance. If cooperation improves the facility's financial health, the union may use the negotiation process to obtain its share. It seems therefore that unions are in a good position to assure themselves the fruits of cooperation. Besides, any management sophisticated enough to overcome years of emotional "hangups" about unions is likely to be smart enough to realize that a sincere effort at cooperation is the only meaningful alternative to threats of strikes and other disruptions.

Nevertheless a lack of sensitivity on labor's part to the situation faced by managers can undermine attempts at cooperation. Union leaders and members must be aware of the following:

1. Management's need for efficiency and effectiveness.
2. The image held of unions by managers.
3. Precedents set by practice.

Management's Efficiency and Effectiveness

Managers are evaluated, rewarded, and promoted largely on the basis of how well they perform. This means that managers must be efficient and effective. Efficiency means accomplishing objectives with a minimum of resources and in a timely manner. The desire for efficiency can cause managers at all levels to react negatively to union work rules and jurisdictional standards. Managers are uniformly indifferent to who does what. They are more concerned with what gets done. In the pursuit of efficiency an administrator may assign a member of the bargaining unit to do some task that should be performed by an employee with a different job description. At times supervisors may do work themselves that should be handled by a rank-and-file member. Union leaders see such actions as administrative indifference to the labor agreement. The supervisor may be simply pursuing goals of efficiency and not intentionally violating the agreement [5].

If the transgression of the contract is important, a grievance should be filed. If a grievance is being filed merely out of resentment, however, the union leader should question the benefits of escalation. Escalation forces both sides into a defensive posture. Efforts become focused upon *how* things are done and not *what* is done, and efficiency suffers. The less efficient the organization, the smaller the available pool of resources to be divided between workers and the employer.

Escalation also results in a strict interpretation of the rules. Little room is left for implicit agreements between management and the union. When special circumstances do arise, reliance upon a strict interpretation of the contract curtails appropriate concessions and naturally reduces the level of enjoyment associated with the work environment.

Effectiveness is more than just being efficient. A supervisor may be very quick (efficient) to make decisions, but if the decisions are wrong, the manager is ineffective. Ineffective decisions are never efficient, because resources are wasted. If the union adheres to a literal interpretation of the contract, the administrators may be forced to select less effective solutions to situations simply because of potential union reaction to more effective alternatives. For example, if the most effective order requires a nurse to make an adjustment on a piece of equipment, the supervisor may hesitate to give that order because such work is not the duty of the nurse. The less efficient and less effective solution required might involve sending a requisition to the maintainance department. The labor agreement is followed to the letter, but organizational effectiveness is reduced. One such incident is irrelevant. When hundreds of minor decisions are made every day, however, and each is slightly suboptimal, efficiency and effectiveness suffer. This leads to smaller surplus revenues for wage increases, fringe benefits, holidays, etc.

It is imperative that union officials acknowledge administrators' needs for efficiency and effectiveness without undermining the survival need of the union, its leaders, or its members. Otherwise, the employer *and* the employees ultimately suffer.

Union Image

By the time most potential administrators graduate from college they have formed an opinion of unions. This attitude is often based on incomplete information and reflects the prejudices of parents, peers, and professors. Usually stories of union violence and corruption are generalized to all employee organizations. Strikes and union "make-work" rules add to the negative image of these groups. Given these decidedly unfavorable opinions, even reasonable union actions are often distorted to substantiate many managers' preconceptions. In the minds of administrators, therefore, a union becomes merely another obstacle that must be tolerated.

If the union-management relationship is to grow into one of cooperation, the union must change its image in the eyes of the administrators [6]. The union must come to be viewed as a cooperative contributor to the organization's effectiveness. This is easy to postulate but difficult to implement.

The first step is for the union to evaluate its actions and its reactions to management initiatives. When grievances are being submitted, what is their motivation? Is the union trying to right a wrong or is it merely retaliating against an inconsequential management action? Are stewards and higher officials allowing political grievances to be formalized and thus further confirming management's preconceptions? Are terms sometimes put into the contract just to limit management actions, or do they all have more meaningful motivations? Only the union officials in each labor-management relationship can accurately answer these questions. In exploring them, union leaders must have in mind management's goals of efficiency and effectiveness. If the union can further the objectives that labor and management have in common, its image will slowly change. Cooperation will become an increasingly more realistic alternative in the minds of management.

The other major effort that the union should make is to offer a positive contribution to the organization. Union leaders and workers often see changes or improvements that could be made in the operation of the facility. A common mistake is to inform the supervisor responsible for the area. This may make the supervisor resentful, since suggestions are an implicit form of criticism. A suggestion system established *within* the union allows ideas to be evaluated in terms of how members would be affected. Suggestions that offer a meaningful improvement in efficiency or effectiveness can be suggested to top administrators by the union leaders. Many of the ideas may be unworkable for reasons of which the union is unaware. Those that do hold promise have the advantage, in management's view, of being supported by the employee organization. Thus, the union can help the administrators to do a better job. This should not be the union's primary concern, but the establishment of a suggestion committee costs nothing and the gains can be substantial to the employer. Astute negotiators will see that some of the savings due to these suggestions accrue to the workers in the form of better contract settlements.

If the benefits of a more enjoyable work environment and improved contracts are to be obtained, the union must minimize interruptions to management effectiveness and efficiency. At the same time the employee organization should make a meaningful, positive contribution to the employer. Nothing in the labor laws requires such actions, and many union leaders who have unsuccessfully tried to create a cooperative atmosphere would argue that such efforts are a waste of time. Nevertheless what are the alternatives? Resentment? Open hostility? Who benefits from a belligerent environment?

Precedents

A final word of caution concerns precedents. If management is allowed to undertake an action prohibited by the contract, the union may lose the ability to prevent it in the future. Extracontractual activities by management must be scrutinized by union leaders. Should administrators violate the agreement or past precedents and the union fail to declare a grievance, the employer will have a defense against future grievances on the issue. Arbitrators are very sympathetic to the argument that no complaint was registered when the same action was undertaken previously. For example, suppose the agreement requires that all subcontracting be discussed with the union. The administrators decide to paint the building without consulting the union. In a spirit of cooperation the union does not file a complaint, since none of the union members are affected. Next, management decides to subcontract an addition to the parking lot without consulting the employee organization. Again, union members are not harmed, and no grievance is filed. Finally, management decides to subcontract food preparation. The union files a grievance because it was not consulted. Management denies the complaint on the basis that the union had waived (by its past inactions) the right to be consulted. The arbitration decision may go in favor of the union, but the management argument is carefully considered and may control the final decision.

This does not mean the union should try to stop every management decision. When a decision affects contractual rights, the union should complain formally to protect its rights. The complaint may be filed with management and then conceded in the case of the painting or parking lot examples. When a critical issue does come up, however, it can be shown that the union has not waived its rights. There is a delicate balance between protecting rights and filing grievances simply to harass management. To avoid destroying cooperation and still maintain contractual rights, a grievance should be filed according to the following procedures. At the time it is filed, the reason for the formal complaint is explained and the need for protecting future rights pointed out. If the case at hand has no impact on the employee organization, it is promptly conceded. This illustrates to management that the union wishes to cooperate and at the same time puts the labor organization on record as not waiving its rights.

COOPERATION THROUGH CONSULTATION

Cooperation is largely a matter of consultation of each side by the other. Most resentment arises because one party has not been informed of the motivations behind the other's actions. In such cases it is only reasonable that motivations will be inferred from past behavior. When the relationship between labor and management is young, inferences are based upon previously held conceptions. Too often these are misconceptions. Even in mature relationships, past experiences leave room to question present actions.

Proactive vs. Reactive Stance

Each phase of collective action finds one party primarily on the defensive and the other primarily on the offensive. In organizing, the union takes the offensive; that is, the union is proactive. It is the organizers who decide when to solicit signatures openly or to request an election. Management, by the nature of the situation, is forced into a defensive or reactive role; it must react to the union's actions. Contract negotiations follow much the same pattern. The employee organization makes demands, and administrators are forced to defend their positions. In both organizing and negotiations, management can assume the offensive temporarily through careful planning. Well-conceived personnel policies coupled with fair treatment leave the collective action group few areas in which to take the offensive. Likewise, sound counterproposals can take the initiative away from the union in contract negotiations. When the union makes demands and management makes a counteroffer, the employee representatives must defend their original demand.

In contract administration the roles are reversed. Normally it is management that is on the offensive and the union that is on the defensive. Management makes decisions and takes action. The union typically accepts the results or must oppose them by filing a grievance. In rare cases the union may gain the initiative by submitting positive suggestions. However, since it is management that is responsible for the operation of the facility, union initiatives are short-lived.

These traditional scenarios are based upon a reactive model of labor relations: one side acts, the other reacts. Each side makes its positive contribution before any action is taken. Through consultation engaged in before any action is carried out, the environment can become proactive. Not only does participation lead to a greater commitment to the success of new undertakings, it facilitates cooperation, since each party understands the motivations underlying the proposed actions.

The proactive approach is primarily related to contract administration, although it can be applied to contract negotiations. If open communications are maintained between labor and management during the administrative phase of labor relations, the topics in negotiations are well known before discussions begin [3]. Each side already knows the principal concerns of the other. Surprises, which can lead to strikes, are minimized. If consultation is consistently practiced in the administration of the contract, cooperation is increased. When negotiations are undertaken, compromises are more frequent. Each side realizes that the other is pursuing positive goals and not merely trying to undermine the other.

Consultation has other direct benefits. Managers find that the implementation of changes is met with union support, not resistance. If the appropriate union official is aware of a proposed change and the reasons for it, there is no need for the official to obstruct the project just to assert leadership. Participation modifies the perspective of those involved. When a union leader can make suggestions that are accepted, a proposal becomes "our" idea and not just "management's." Through the informal organization — the grapevine — the union leader can work *for* the concept with members. The motivation to do so comes in large part from the leader's change in perspective. Like most people, union leaders like to see "their" ideas implemented. Consultation benefits the union leaders in that they are looked to for information by the rank and file. When the leaders are on the inside of the management decision-making process, they are more knowledgeable. They have more to offer the members. This additional knowledge serves to enhance the leaders' power and helps assure their reelection and control over dissident groups within the local [7]. The result is a more stable union organization.

Cooperation through consultation, therefore, benefits the employer, the union, its leaders, and its members. It is truly a positive approach to labor relations. Unfortunately misconceptions and past differences make it difficult for either side to initiate cooperation.

IMPLEMENTING COOPERATION

Countless factors contribute to the mistrust that commonly exists between union and management officials. To change the employment environment into a cooperative one is a difficult task. If the task is not undertaken, however, labor-management relations can become a detriment to the effective delivery of health care. Through cooperation, new opportunities to provide better service to clients is possible.

There is no one best way to undertake the long journey toward cooperation. Sometimes the first step is made when one side is in a desperate situation and needs a favor. When favors are granted, they carry with them the implied expectation of reciprocation. If returned, simple requests may slowly grow into a cooperative relationship. Unfortunately waiting for such opportunities does not assure they will occur, nor do such opportunities guarantee a favorable relationship. Positive action is needed.

One technique already mentioned is for the union to make constructive suggestions to help management. Whether these ideas result from a formal suggestion system within the union or from observations of union leaders does not matter. It is a positive step.

Another area for establishing cooperation is in labor relations training. Many organizations and unions undertake some form of training to inform supervisors and stewards of new changes in the contract. Usually these efforts are carried out independently. In the name of reducing grievances management might suggest that the training be done jointly at management's expense. Since the nominal purpose is to train employees — both supervisors and workers — in the meaning of the contract, the training can properly be done at management's expense without constituting a labor law violation of union domination. The union does not lose, since the training results in the stewards' being paid while they learn rather than being instructed in their free time. Of course the trainers include a representative of the employer and of the union; the purpose of the training is training, not indoctrination.

There are several gains from this joint training. First, misinterpretations of the contract held by union or management trainers will not be perpetuated. Ideally the trainers can work out instructional plans together, and resolve misunderstandings before the training sessions start. Second, since stewards and supervisors are given the same presentation at the same time, grievances resulting from simple misconceptions are likely to be diminished. Third, if the stewards and supervisors observe higher level union and management officials cooperating in the explanation of the contract, they have a model to follow when the lower level union and management members must interact [8].

The training may be nothing more sophisticated than allowing union and management representatives to take turns reading and paraphrasing the contract. This causes the stewards and supervisors to see that there is one interpretation for each provision of the agreement.

Other joint efforts are also possible. Clubs, interest groups, athletic leagues, and charity drives can be jointly sponsored. The object of these cooperative efforts is secondary in importance to the experience gained by mutually satisfying interactions — interactions that allow each side to reassess its opinion of the other and build confidence in the possibility of teamwork.

LABOR RELATIONS PHILOSOPHY

Providers should attempt to develop a reasonable philosophy of labor relations. That philosophy must recognize the needs of all parties — labor, management, and the public. Personal interests cannot be ignored in favor of the needs of the employer or labor organization. Some components of a labor relations philosophy are listed below. Other dimensions should be added by each provider to reflect the unique relationship of his or her particular situation.

1. The survival of the employer is paramount. Without the health care facility, the need for an employee organization is nonexistent.
2. Administrators at all levels must recognize the survival needs of the union, its leaders, and its members. All management actions should consider the implications of these survival needs.
3. Workers and union leaders must respect the employer's need for efficiency and effectiveness.
4. Problem solving should be undertaken jointly with a pragmatic and not an ideological viewpoint.
5. Cooperation is the most viable long-term strategy for all parties. It is the only means through which the delivery of health care is improved.

SUMMARY

The success of labor-management relations depends upon cooperation. For cooperation to work, each side must view the labor relationship as one in which each can benefit by helping the other. The traditional adversary approach is strongly embodied in labor laws and past practices. Overcoming this tradition requires overcoming stereotyped thinking, mistrust, and resentment. Union leaders must realize that the more effectively management can manage, the greater will be the potential benefits to the employees. Likewise, management must look upon the union and its leaders as allies, not enemies.

Management must not rush into cooperation with such vigor that it dominates the union. In dealing with the employee organization it is important for administrators to remember that the union as an organization has *survival needs,* as do its leaders and its members. Management actions that threaten any of these will be met by strong resistance. Likewise the union is a *political* institution, and its leaders politicians. Before evaluating actions by the employee organization it is important to realize that the motivations may be solely political. Irrespective of the nature of the relationship, *precedents* can effectively change the intent of the contract. Care should be exercised not to permit variations from accepted policies without comment.

Union leaders must be careful not to undermine their credibility with members by appearing too cooperative toward management. These leaders must also be aware of management's desire for effectiveness and efficiency. Many actions that appear to be antiunion moves are simply attempts by the administration to make the facility more effective. The image of unions is generally unfavorable among managers. The union can overcome this only through a careful screening of grievances and positive contributions to the well-being of the employer. Unions, too, must be sensitive to the problem of precedents. Failure to protect contract terms may cause those terms to become inoperative.

If labor and management are to develop a better working relationship, the framework in which they operate will have to evolve from a reactive to a proactive approach. Each side must consult the other before taking action. Unilateral action merely confirms past suspicions and negative images held by the other side.

POINTS FOR REFLECTION

1. What is a zero-sum relationship as opposed to a positive relationship?
2. What precautions must management exercise in its cooperation with unions?
3. How do precautions that the union should exercise compare with those of management?
4. Describe proactive and reactive labor relations.
5. How can cooperation between management and union be implemented?

SELECTED READINGS

1. Crockett, William J. The management conflict with democratic values. *Business Horizons* 16:13, 1973.
2. Deloughery, Grace L., and Kristine M. Gebbie. *Political Dynamics: Impact on Nurses and Nursing.* Saint Louis: C. V. Mosby Company, 1975.

3. Golightly, Henry O.   The what, what not, and how of internal communications. *Business Horizons* 16:13, 1973.
4. Longest, Beaufort B., and Donald E. Clawson.   The effect of selected turnover factors on hospital turnover rates. *Personnel Journal* 53:30, 1974.
5. Nash, Al.   Hospital values, conflicts, and supervisory practices. *Personnel Journal* 52:1056, 1973.
6. Sloane, Arthur A.   Unions and union imagery. *Personnel Journal* 52:470, 1973.
7. Thompsom, Duane E., and Richard P. Borglum.   A case study of employee attitudes and labor unrest. *Industrial and Labor Relations Review* 27:74, 1973.
8. Werther, William B., Jr.   Reducing grievances through effective contract administration. *Labor Law Journal* 25:211, 1974.
9. White, J. Kenneth, and Robert A. Ruh.   Effects of personal values on the relationship between participation and job attitudes. *Administrative Science Quarterly* 18:506, 1973.

11

Emergent Forces in Labor Relations

*We demand that big business give the people a square deal: in return
we must insist that when any one engaged in big business honestly en-
deavors to do right he shall himself be given a square deal.*
                                                    — *Theodore Roosevelt*

The future course of labor relations in the health care industry will
be an evolutionary one. It will be an extension of present developments
with few radical changes. There will be no nationwide rush toward or
away from collective action. Some employers have already been organized, others will be in the future, and still others never will be unionized.
The outcome for individual institutions and for the entire health care
industry depends upon a confluence of forces [13]. The two most obvious
and strongest ones are the increasing acceptance of unionization and the
increasing sophistication of administrators. Each partially offsets the
other.

UNIONS

Unions are gaining acceptance among a wide range of professions.
Doctors, nurses, teachers, athletes, actors, police, musicians, and many
other diverse occupations have some degree of unionization. Collective
action is no longer limited to blue-collar workers, if it ever was. The
nonprofessional stigma associated with unions is fading. As health care
employees see professionals forming unions and read about large contract settlements, collective action will appear a pragmatic (if not always

agreeable) solution. In the future the individual's decision to pursue collective action will be based less on emotionalism and more upon the realities of the situation. "Am I being treated fairly by supervision?" "Is the organization taking care of my interests?" These and other questions will evoke the answers that determine unionization.

As unionization is becoming more acceptable to workers, administrators are also becoming more sophisticated in dealing with employees. Modernized personnel policies, supervisory training in labor relations, and the realization that the health care organization's most important resource is its people have led to an improved working environment in many facilities. In those institutions that have failed to implement changes, unions have appeared, or will shortly. Unionization will continue to become more acceptable as management becomes more capable and feels more comfortable in dealing with unions.

A number of developments other than unionization will influence the shape of labor-management relations in the health care field. Some are within the control of providers, and others are beyond the purview of the labor-management relationship. Providers must assess these developments in terms of their consequences for management, employees, and clients.

LEGISLATION

For years proprietary and nonprofit health care institutions were treated separately from other employers under employment-related laws. This difference is blurring as Congress slowly moves toward the position that, if an employee-related law is good in one sector, it should be applied to all employment relationships. The last exceptions to this position are state employees and managers.

State employees will be covered sooner or later by federal labor laws. It does not matter whether this coverage results from legislation or from a ruling by the Supreme Court that all citizens should have equal protection under the law. When the change occurs, state and county hospital administrators will be forced to undergo the same transition that nonprofit health care administrators did in the mid-1970's. Furthermore, state and county public health departments will be confronted for the first time with union activity that possesses legal power.

The extension of labor laws to supervisors and middle managers would have even more of an impact. Although these classifications are specifically excluded in the health care industry (and in other industries), top management's neglect and abuse of this group may well result in a change in their status. Unless actions are taken to provide more security for middle and lower level managers, top management's link to the workers will be unionized. In fact nothing in the labor laws prevents these managerial levels from forming unions today, but because this group is not covered by the law, top administrators are free to discriminate against managers who join or support collective action [10]. Lack of power and protection for middle and lower level managers creates a security gap [12] which, if ignored long enough, and if abuses become glaring, will be taken care of by legislative or judicial action.

Other legislative changes are also probable. The last four decades have shown that new laws designed to influence the employment relationship occur every few years. The National Labor Relations Act, Social Security Act, Fair Labor Standards Act, Taft-Hartley Act, Welfare Pension Plans Disclosure Act, Landrum-Griffin Act, Civil Rights Act, Occupational Safety and Health Act, Nonprofit Health Care Amendments to the Labor Management Relations Act, and Employee Retirement Income Security Act are some of the more obvious examples. These laws have been amended and will be amended in the future, and new laws will be designed to assure even more rights to workers. Unless the health care industry corrects its own labor relations abuses as they are identified, legislation will be enacted to take care of them. Organizations that have alleviated sources of maltreatment will find compliance a simple matter. Otherwise, panic and inefficiency will ensue as the employer attempts to comply with new legal mandates [8].

Nationwide medical care will also receive legislative action in the immediately foreseeable future. Whether this action will follow the European model of socialized medicine or will be an extension of the private enterprise system through insurance carriers is uncertain. Nevertheless it is obvious that citizens in the United States spend a disproportionately high amount of their personal income for medical care when compared with other industrial nations. For all the talk about patient care and advanced technologies, informed providers know that other nations provide statistically better medical care for more of the population and do it at a lower per capita cost. The problem is not a lack of ability among American providers. It is that the system of health care delivery provides superb care only to those who can afford it.

Legislation enacted to provide health care to all the public will bring controls, reporting requirements, and demands for evaluation of services offered. Specialization, quotas, standardization, and evaluation will cause a wider application of industrial techniques in an attempt to maximize effectiveness and efficiency while minimizing cost. Unfortunately the routinization of health care may cause increased problems of morale, turnover, and motivation for the facility without an accompanying increase in the quality of care.

Another area ripe for legislative enactments is that of fringe benefits. The federal government has regulated the minimum wage since the 1930's, but fringe benefits are an area in which few laws have been passed. The Employee Retirement Income Security Act in 1974, however, may signal a new era. For the increasingly espoused purpose of achieving a smaller federal bureaucracy, politicians will turn to employers to implement improvements for workers. Medical insurance, for example, may well be accomplished by forcing employers to provide minimum insurance levels for employees. If this happens — and health maintenance legislation is an indication that it will — can other federally mandated benefits be far behind? The pension reform law of 1974 could be amended in a few years to guarantee a minimum retirement benefit for all workers. This may be an alternative if the Social Security Administration encounters serious problems in providing benefits as a result of its underlying actuarial assumptions. Time-off benefits, legal insurance, mental health insurance, disability insurance, life insurance, and other mandated fringe benefits would not be far behind.

INFLUENCE OF NONPROFESSIONALS

Nonprofessionals in health care are a group too frequently overlooked by administrators. Future employment growth will occur primarily among these groups. With no professional identification and only an indirect role in patient care, these workers are not going to be satisfied with humanitarian or professional appeals. Increasingly the quality of supervision, wages, and benefits will be the primary determinants of their desire to unionize, since there will be little special dedication to their occupation or employer. It is this group that will carry out the most militant actions, if organized. Moreover its gains will be observed by other employee groups, who will also become activist if they perceive that they are not being given relatively fair treatment.

ASSOCIATIONS AND UNIONS

The conflict between professional associations and unions will concern providers for years. Its dimensions are several. First, health care professionals — whether workers, coordinators, or administrators — need professional associations to keep them up to date in their profession. Second, the labor laws and the employer's need for solidarity dictate that members of management cannot also be members of a group that represents the employees in their dealings with the employer. Third, the viability of many professional associations will be determined by how well the association can emulate the role of a union. Fourth, unions of professionals will have to be concerned with the professionals' development.

Some of these dimensions are at present mutually exclusive. A union cannot possibly meet the needs of all professionals, because manager-professionals must be excluded. On the other hand, if a professional association attempts to represent members through collective bargaining, manager-professionals will have to resign from it, too. In some areas, however, the professional association will atrophy and disappear if it does not actively represent those bargaining units that seek representation.

One tactic is for the professional associations to divide themselves internally into two divisions — one concerned with bargaining and the other with professionalism. Unless the NLRB and employers are willing to recognize this distinction, the move will do little more than dilute the associations' resources. The other alternative is to declare their intent one way or the other. Whichever route is elected — union representation or professional advancement — a void will be created. If the association retains its professional purpose exclusively, the organizing of providers will be left to the more traditional unions. Although both the professional association and the unions will coexist, it is likely that the union will become the dominant force in every encounter. The union will make the meaningful changes in the work environment and will become the source of power and income. Professional associations will eventually decline in size and importance.

The other alternative is for the professional associations to become unions. Union security clauses and positive improvements for the members will assure their survival, even if in a much altered form. Manager-professionals will experience a void in professional development which unions will not be able to fill. The result will be a much greater demand on educational institutions, private seminars, and conferences to provide continuing education.

Each of these alternatives holds significant implications for providers. The concerned professional stands to lose the opportunity for growth afforded by the professional association — either because the importance of the association will decline or because professionals will lose membership once they reach a supervisory position. Administrators stand to lose because of an increased reluctance of professionals to abandon membership in the association as the quid pro quo of a managerial role. Even when the trade-off is accepted, the employer loses because of the increased difficulty for manager-professionals to remain professionally informed and up to date.

WOMEN'S CONSCIOUSNESS

Anyone who has watched television or read a newspaper knows the roles of women are undergoing a rapid reformulation. The stereotyped view of a female nurse or technologist as a docile, subservient employee is increasingly unrealistic. More and more women are heads of households and work out of necessity; a higher percentage realize that assertiveness is the only way to obtain more for themselves [7]. The connection between individual assertiveness and group action is obvious. Group action makes individual efforts more powerful. The actions of California Nurses' Association in the San Francisco Bay area provide an appropriate example of how far-reaching this new consciousness and group action can be.

TRENDS IN COMMUNITY HEALTH

The trend toward moving health care closer to the client also has consequences for industrial relations. As health care is decentralized, there will be a proliferation of small clinics and hospitals. These may be part of, or affiliated with, larger health care systems. Organizing a facility with several thousand employees is generally more costly than organizing smaller units. If the NLRB considers these smaller facilities appropriate bargaining units, the administrators of the entire system may face a multitude of contracts and personnel policies. Inevitably this leads to inequities and criticism. Smaller facilities may become the "crack in the armor" that leads to the entire system's being organized. Even if system-wide organization does not result, the administrative function will become considerably more complex.

EDUCATIONAL CHANGES

Unionization in the health care field means that continuing education among managers will have a new dimension. Not only must advanced management techniques be learned, but rapid legal and social changes related to unions cause labor relations to be a continuously evolving field that must be constantly studied. Techniques that are permissible one day can become illegal the next as a result of a court or NLRB decision. Seminars, reading, and a careful studying of weekly labor reports will be necessary to stay informed [11].

The problems precipitated by unionization will lead to a change in educational institutions, too. Within a few years administrators should be able to find recent graduates who are better informed in labor and human relations techniques. The emphasis in nursing, hospital administration, and other health care—related curricula will change. More importance will be placed on people-related management skills, even at the expense of administrative techniques such as budgeting, planning, and organizing.

Admittedly, other trends will shape the roles of all providers in the area of labor relations. Many of these forces will be made explicit through the process of collective bargaining [11].

BARGAINING TRENDS

Some of the changes that will be imposed upon providers by outside forces such as clients, technological improvements, governmental rulings and laws, the economy, and community expectations have already been touched upon. Even more changes, however, will be imposed by each party on the other through the collective bargaining relationship. These changes will directly influence the behavior of management, the union, and the employees. The most prominent topics of collective bargaining will be union security, fringe benefits, wages, resolution of grievances, and professional standards.

Union Security

If employees feel strongly enough to form a union, the issue of union security will be a high-priority item. In states that permit it, the labor organization will strive for a union shop clause that requires all bargaining unit members to join the union. The checkoff — an arrangement by which management deducts dues and remits them to the union — will be another goal in union security.

Although union security provisions entrench the employee organization within the facility, they do provide benefits for everyone. The security provision allows union leaders greater flexibility in cooperating with management. The energies devoted to constantly recruiting new employees can be diverted to assisting with beneficial changes. Since, under a union shop clause, everyone must belong, the leaders need not consider the effects of their actions on prospective members. Political considerations still exist within the union, but if meaningful improvements are made, criticism from upstarts has a much diluted impact. Employees benefit in that the cost of operating the union is shared.

Fringe Benefits

Fringe benefits are the fastest-growing component of labor costs. Part of the reason for this trend is that they are largely inflation-proof. If the employer pays all of each employee's health insurance, the employees are unaffected as the costs of these premiums rise. Another inflation-proof benefit is time-off with pay. The value to the worker of an extra day off is unchanged by the inflation rate, although cost to the employer may increase rapidly.

Fringe benefits also have tax advantages for employees. For example, if a life insurance policy costs $200 a year, the employee might have to earn $240 before taxes to have enough after-tax money to pay for the policy. When the employer agrees to pay for the policy, it is as if the employee received a $240, before taxes, raise. The true cost to the employer is in fact probably much less. First, the employer may secure a group policy, which can reduce the average cost per policy to $150. In addition the policy is paid with *before*-tax dollars in the case of a proprietary institution. The entire $150 per employee is deducted as a business expense. Only after these outlays are deducted from income is the remainder (profit) taxed. If the employer is in a 50 percent tax bracket, profits are reduced by $75 per employee. The true after-tax cost to the employer is $75, whereas it would cost an employee $240 of pre-tax earnings. This arrangement in the tax laws has helped the rapid proliferation of fringe benefits in the post–World War II period [9].

The problem with fringe benefits is the question, "What does the employer gain?" For a long time the argument was that the employer remained competitive in the labor market. Actually most employees cannot recite — let alone understand — their benefits and are therefore influenced very little by them [3]. This poor return to the employer, coupled with a rapid increase in the cost of benefits, is leading to a re-examination of the use of fringe benefits.

One alternative is for more organizations to go toward a flexible fringe-benefit program. Under this program, which has serious tax complications, each worker is given an account equal to the amount the organization now spends on benefits. The employee then "buys" benefits against this employer-held account. This leads to a greater recognition of what benefits are being received and permits optimal use of money spent and optimal satisfaction of needs. Younger employees can obtain comprehensive life and medical insurance, while older workers can choose larger contributions to medical insurance and their retirement fund. Under traditional benefit programs younger and older workers form pressure groups within the organization (or union) to have benefits improved on a wide front. Why not? If management will expand benefits for employees and pay the tab, the benefits are free to the workers. Under flexible benefits, the trade-offs are made by the employees, with each self-designed benefit package providing higher worker satisfaction [9].

Wages

Excluding some highly paid professionals, the health care industry has historically paid low wages. This happened partly because the employees were seen as deriving satisfaction from helping their fellow man and partly to keep the cost of health care down. Collective action is going to force even small employers to utilize modern wage and salary techniques. Wages will have to be comparable to those in jobs outside the health care industry, while relative wages within an institution will have to be more closely related to the responsibilities and abilities of the workers.

Administrative failure to bring wages into line with reality will be a source of strength for union organizers and a major issue of contention between bargainers. Undoubtedly wages will go up. Profit and nonprofit institutions will pass the costs on to society. An outraged public and politicians will demand increased government control. This will lead to an increased concern over productivity. Attempts will be made to relate wage increases to productivity gains, since this is the only way to reduce the inflationary impact of growing labor costs. For example, if every employee were suddenly 10 percent more productive, a 10 percent wage increase would not increase costs. Unfortunately theorists are only beginning to understand the complexities of worker productivity [5]. If it could be measured accurately, most collectively bargained wage increases would depend on improvements in productivity. Inflation would become a topic in history and not one in economics [13].

Resolving Grievances

Contract negotiations will focus on dispute resolution. There is probably no greater service provided by a union than an effective grievance system. Union leaders realize this. Contract negotiators will find that resolution of grievances is an ongoing issue that is never completely settled.

The history of success with grievances in the industrial sector has led to fairly standardized grievance mechanisms. Complaints are discussed between labor and management counterparts until an agreement is reached or until top officials are involved. When a satisfactory solution is not forthcoming, arbitration is the normal conclusion. Although refinements will be made, the major trend in this area will be to extend the use of arbitration to virtually every conceivable source of disputes [11].

Professional Standards

Labor-management relations in the industrial sector has seldom had to deal with professional issues, and some administrators are hesitant or reluctant to begin to include them in negotiations. Except in the educational field, there is only limited knowledge and experience of how to handle professional issues in labor-management relations. The inclusion of the health care industry under the NLRA markedly increases the number of potential professionals who will be represented in collective action. The professional, almost by definition, is as concerned with the issues of professional practice as with wages, hours, and working conditions. As more and more professionals join in collective action, administrators will be forced to deal with more of these issues.

Professional concerns also provide a rallying point behind which public support can be won or lost for the employees and the union. If the care offered does not ensure the safety and well-being of the client, the professional may choose to demand negotiation over a method of guaranteeing a more consistent level of care. If a strike is called to force the issue, the public may see only the unstaffed health care facility. The anger and fear generated by this may outweigh the professional's appeal for support to bring better quality care to the public. The longer term goal of the professional may be excellent, but to the individual needing health care, a hospital without staff is a cause for resentment. Conversely, should management be the one causing a continued strike or lockout, public resentment can turn against the health care employer.

As issues of professional concern reach the bargaining table, inaction on the part of either management or the professional employees may bring legislative involvement. Professional standards would then be mandated nationwide and little room for adjustment deemed necessary in individual health care facilities.

Attention to professional issues in contract negotiations may result in new and varied training sections for professionals, more staff, educational leaves, and other changes, each of which increases costs. Passing these costs on to the public does little to enhance the image of an institution. When the professionals' demands are pointed to as the cause for increases, professionals must be able to demonstrate the benefits that accrue to the facility and the public. If they are unable to demonstrate these benefits, the validity of their existence and special needs will be questioned.

Given the complexity of these issues, it is foolish to attempt to resolve them in only a few weeks of talks at the bargaining table. Decisions made hastily under pressure for a settlement and because of other urgent topics can lead to higher costs or inappropriate care patterns. A more reasonable approach is to establish joint study committees formed of high level administrators and employee representatives. (This can be done whether a union is present or not.) Topics related to care can be discussed and given careful consideration, after which recommendations can be made. To the extent that they are mutually acceptable, these suggestions can be formalized by inclusion in the labor-management agreement. An equitable resolution of such issues is possible only through joint, participatory study.

COLLECTIVE ACTION

The need for collective action is not a problem but a symptom — a symptom of oversight by the employer. It may be simplistic, but employers get the type of union they deserve. Those administrators that develop sound policies, carefully consider the economic and personal needs of the employees, provide good working conditions, use well-trained supervisors, and support a meaningful grievance procedure will find that the possibility of unionization is minimal. What could the union offer workers under these ideal circumstances? Health care facilities that do not attend to *all* these basic areas force employees into a trap. Employees can stay and accept the unpleasant aspect of the work environment; they can leave and give up friendships and accumulated benefits and start all over; or they can seek redress from management via the intervention of a third party. It does not really matter whether that third party is a professional association or a union. Each will behave in a way designed to further the well-being of the employee organization, its leaders, and its members.

The federal government has provided a detailed body of law and specific procedures designed to ensure that workers can obtain equity if their work environment is not satisfactory. The need to resort to those procedures should be viewed by management as a failure to maintain its human resources effectively. *It is not a matter of whether employees should or should not join unions. It is a question of whether management is doing its job correctly.*

The burden falls upon administrators, because they have the power. Management decides how resources are allocated and how people are treated. The employer has the authority to right wrongs before they open a schism between the organization's objectives and the objectives of the employees. When management fails in its responsibility, labor laws, outsiders, and agitators cannot be blamed for the resulting unionization of the work force. The blame is squarely with management; it comes with the territory.

There is a management axiom that succinctly summarizes this viewpoint. It is appropriately called the "Iron Law of Responsibility." It states, "In the long run, those who do not use power in a manner which society considers responsible will tend to lose it" [1].

Management and employees in the health care field both have power. How they use it will determine the future of labor-management relations in this industry. More importantly, the use of this power will determine the quality of health care in the United States.

POINTS FOR REFLECTIONS

1. What are the major trends discussed in this chapter?
2. What are the implications of these trends for *today's* labor-management relations?
3. What trends not discussed in this chapter will influence the delivery of health care?
4. What trends not discussed in this chapter will influence labor-management relations in the health care field?

SELECTED READINGS

1. Davis, Keith, and Robert L. Blomstrom. *Business Society and Environment: Social Power and Social Response* (3rd ed.). New York: McGraw-Hill Book Company, 1975.
2. Deloughery, Grace L., and Kristine M. Gebbie. *Political Dynamics: Impact on Nurses and Nursing.* St. Louis: C. V. Mosby Company, 1975.
3. Holey, William H., Jr., and Earl Ingram II. Communicating fringe benefits. *The Personnel Administrator* 18:22, 1973.
4. Kerr, Clark. Educational Changes: Potential Impact on Industrial Relations. In Gerald G. Somers (Ed.), *The Next Twenty-Five Years of Industrial Relations.* Madison, Wisconsin: Industrial Relations Research Association, 1973.
5. Ruch, William A., and James C. Hershauer. *Factors Affecting Worker*

Productivity. Tempe, Arizona: Bureau of Business & Economic Research, College of Business Administration, Arizona State University, 1974.
6. Thompson, Mark. Applying a theory of the future of industrial relations to North America. *Labor Law Journal* 24:563, 1973.
7. Raphael, Edna E. Working women and their membership in labor unions. *Monthly Labor Review* 97:27, 1974.
8. Werther, William B., Jr. Government control v. corporate ingenuity. *Labor Law Journal* 26:360, 1975.
9. Werther, William B., Jr. A new direction in rethinking fringe benefits. *MSU Business Topics* 22:35, 1974.
10. Werther, William B., Jr. Reducing grievances through effective contract administration. *Labor Law Journal* 25:211, 1974.
11. Werther, William B., Jr. Labor relations: Current trend and the future. *Arizona Business* 21:11, 1974.
12. Wright, Robert G. Managing management resources through corporation constitutionalism. *Human Resource Management* 12:13, 1973.
13. Young, Edwin. Personnel Relations in Non-Profit Institutions. In Gerald G. Somers (Ed.), *The Next Twenty-Five Years of Industrial Relations.* Madison, Wisconsin: Industrial Relations Research Association, 1973.

Glossary

administrative law judge An employee of the National Labor Relations Board who presides over and renders decisions in unfair labor practice hearings.

affirmative action program Employer's plan for ensuring equal and fair treatment for people of any race, religion, sex, or national origin.

affirmative order A directive issued by a labor relations board to parties found to have engaged in unfair labor practices, instructing them to undo the effect of such practices so far as possible.

AFL-CIO See American Federation of Labor and Congress of Industrial Organizations

Age Discrimination in Employment Act A 1967 law enforced by the United States Department of Labor to ensure that covered organizations do not discriminate on the basis of age against those forty to sixty-five years old.

agency shop An agreement whereby nonunion members must pay the representative union a sum equal to union dues but need not actually join the union.

Alliance for Labor Action An alliance between the Teamsters and the Auto Workers unions with the goal of organizing unorganized workers.

American Arbitration Association (AAA) A nonprofit, nonpartisan group that serves the labor relations community by providing professional arbitrators and mediators. The Association also provides fact-finders and conducts expedited arbitration.

American Federation of Labor and Congress of Industrial Organizations The major association of unions in the United States. It is responsible for representing organized labor's views on national issues. It was formed in 1955 by a merger of the AFL and the CIO.

Anti-Strikebreaking Act A federal law forbidding the interstate transportation of strikebreakers.

arbitration The use of an impartial third party to break an impasse. A decision rendered by an arbitrator is final and binding on both parties.

attrition principle An agreement to reduce the number of jobs existing in an industry solely by normal employee turnover (such as resignations, deaths, and retirements).

authorization card A card or petition signed by an employee to indicate a desire to have an election to determine whether a union will be designated as the employee's bargaining agent.

Board That part of the National Labor Relations Board which is responsible for administering the judicial role of the NLRB. The five members serve to review the decisions of administrative law judges.

bargaining agent An organization accepted by the employer or certified by a government agency as the representative of all bargaining unit employees for the purpose of collective bargaining.

bargaining unit The group of employees accepted by an employer or designated by an authorized agency for the purpose of bargaining collectively regarding their employment conditions.

bill of rights for union members Unofficial term for Title I of the 1959 Labor-Management Reporting and Disclosure Act, which sets forth the rights to which all union members are entitled.

boycott A refusal to buy products from, service, or otherwise deal with an organization.

Byrnes Act *See* Anti-Strikebreaking Act.

cease-and-desist order A decree by the National Labor Relations Board directing a party to curtail an action that is deemed an unfair labor practice.

certification The official designation, by a labor board, of an employee organization as the exclusive bargaining agent for employees of a specified bargaining unit.

certification election An employee vote, decided by the rule of the majority, to determine whether employees within a designated bargaining unit wish an employee organization to act as their exclusive representative in collective bargaining.

charge A written allegation, presented to the National Labor Relations Board, which accuses a certain party of violating the labor laws.

check-off An agreement whereby an employer automatically deducts union dues from employees' pay and remits the dues to the union. For the practice to be legal, a written authorization from each employee must be filed with the employer.

client An individual who receives health care services.

closed shop An illegal agreement whereby only members of a certain union may be hired by an employer.

collective action A joint effort of employees directed at their employer in order to obtain a certain concession.

collective bargaining A process by which representatives of employees negotiate with the employer's representatives to procure a signed agreement covering wages, hours, and conditions of employment that is agreeable to both employees and employer.

company union An employee organization developed and/or supported by an employer. It is outlawed by section 8(a)(2) of the National Labor Relations Act.

conciliation An attempt by a third party to pacify and/or accommodate opposing parties in a labor dispute.

consent election An NLRB election agreed to by both labor and management. After all protests are filed (or after five days), the regional director can announce the results of the election. *See also* stipulated election.

contract Written proof of an agreement between two or more parties specifying the wages, hours, and conditions of employment in a work setting.

contract administration The broad process of making the collectively bargained agreement work, so that each party's rights are protected and each party's privileges obtained.

contract bar rules Guidelines used by the NLRB to determine whether an existing contract between an employer and a union prohibits a representation election sought by a rival union.

decertification election An election held in order to determine whether the employees wish to retain their present union.

de facto bargaining Collective bargaining carried on in the absence of any legislation requiring it, usually because of employee and outside pressures.

de minimis rule or doctrine Term used in arbitration to define extremely minor violations or trifling matters of which the law does not take notice.

Douglas doctrine (trilogy cases) The 1960 decision of the United States Supreme Court that whenever a contract permits arbitration, all issues arising from contract administration are subject to arbitration, unless the topic is specifically excluded from arbitration by the contract. This decision also severely limits judicial review of arbitrators' decisions. The three cases involved in the decision were the *United Steelworkers of America* v. *American Manufacturing Company, Warrior and Gulf Navigation Company,* and *Enterprise Wheel and Car Corporation.* Associate Justice Douglas wrote the majority opinion.

dual union An employee organization formed to enlist members from among employees already in another union.

employer association Employers in related enterprises bargaining as a unit with one or more unions.

Equal Employment Opportunity Commission Federal agency that enforces the 1964 Civil Rights Act, as amended, in order to eliminate discrimination on the basis of race, sex, religion, or national origin.

Equal Pay Act A federal act that prohibits the payment of different wages on the basis of the sex of the worker.

escalator clause Contract agreement whereby employee wages rise with the cost of living (generally in relation to the United States Department of Labor's Consumer Price Index — CPI). If the clause has a maximum limit, then it is called a *capped escalator clause.*

Executive Order #11491 (Labor-Management Relations in the Federal Service, October, 1969) Presidential order allowing federal employees to bargain collectively.

expedited arbitration A form of arbitration offered through the American Arbitration Association that concludes with the rendering of a binding decision within a short time relative to traditional arbitration procedures.

Experimental Negotiation Agreement (ENA) An arrangement in the steel industry by which a union foregoes its right to strike at the expiration of the labor contract in exchange for management's promise to provide a token raise and extend new contract terms retroactively to the employees, once a final agreement is reached.

fact-finding board A group of individuals, chosen by a government agency or agreed upon by involved parties, who are delegated to investigate and report on disputed facts.

Fair Labor Standards Act The federal minimum wage law and its amendment *featherbedding* The use of employees in situations in which the work is neither wanted nor needed.

Federal Anti-Injunction Act (Norris-LaGuardia Act) A 1932 law passed to limit the use of federal court injunctions by employers seeking to end strikes or other collective efforts of workers.

Federal Mediation and Conciliation Service (FMCS) Created by the Labor Management Relations Act of 1947 primarily to conciliate and mediate disputes that might erupt into a disruption of interstate commerce. In the health care field the service is empowered to appoint fact-finding boards when contract negotiations may lead to a discontinuation of health care. The FMCS also provides lists of arbitrators and offers steward-foreman training in contract administrations.

final offer arbitration A method of resolving, without a strike, labor-management deadlocks that arise from contract negotiations. The method requires the arbitrator to select whichever offer (union's or management's) is the more reasonable; the arbitrator is constrained to select one proposal or the other and may not create a compromise solution.

fringe benefits Items and services provided employees beyond regular salaries (e.g., pensions, various insurances, and holidays).

good faith bargaining The requirement by the National Labor Relations Act, as interpreted by the National Labor Relations Board, that parties meet at reasonable times to confer in good faith on wages, hours, and conditions of employment. It does not require either party to agree to a proposal or make concessions.

General Counsel (Office of the) That part of the National Labor Relations Board that is responsible for the day-to-day administration of the National Labor Relations Act, as amended. It also supervises the operations of the regional offices.

grievance An allegation by any party functioning under a collective bargaining agreement that a violation of the contract has occurred. Typically this means an employee or union complaint.

grievance committee A group of representatives of the union or management who meet with the other side to resolve grievances.

grievance procedure Established method of adjustment of grievances between parties.

independent union An employee organization that is not affiliated with the American Federation of Labor–Congress of Industrial Organizations or a national union.

industrial union An employee organization that admits all employees in a facility or plant to membership regardless of work performed by a particular employee.

injunction A court order demanding the performance or cessation of specified activities on the grounds that the complaining party will suffer irreparable harm from the activities.

international union A nationally organized union with locals in another country, usually Canada.

jurisdictional dispute A controversy between two employee organizations as to which one has the right to have its members perform a certain type of work.

Labor Management Relations Act (Taft-Hartley Act) The first major amendment (1947) to the National Labor Relations Act. It contained the first statutory prohibitions against unions, exempted nonprofit health care facilities from coverage, and created the Federal Mediation and Conciliation Service.

Labor-Management Reporting and Disclosure Act (Landrum-Griffin Act) An act (1959) modifying the prohibitions established in the National Labor Relations Act and the Labor Management Relations Act. It includes the union members' "Bill of Rights," which sets forth regulations on the behavior of union leaders.

Landrum-Griffin Act See Labor-Management Reporting and Disclosure Act.

local union (local) The smallest organizational division of a union. It normally includes the employees of one employer who have joined together for the purpose of exercising their collective action rights. (In the construction industry, a local usually includes employees within a geographical area who possess a common skill, even though they may work for different employers — e.g., carpenters and plumbers.)

management rights clause (management prerogatives) A clause within the collective bargaining agreement that reserves to management certain rights that are not subject to grievance or arbitration.

master agreement A collective bargaining agreement negotiated with and applicable to more than one institution.

mediator A third party undertaking to propose compromises in order to assist both sides in a dispute to reach an agreement.

mediation-arbitration (Med-Arb) An arrangement whereby an arbitrator attempts to mediate differences between union and management negotiators. Unresolved issues are then decided by the mediator turned arbitrator. This procedure is used to avoid strikes.

National Labor Relations Act (NLRA) (Wagner Act) The first (1935) broad, constitutionally valid, labor relations law. It gave workers wanting to join unions the protection of the federal government, listed unfair labor practices that were prohibited to employers, and created the National Labor Relations Board to enforce the law.

National Labor Relations Board (NLRB) The agency created by the National Labor Relations Act to enforce the act. The NLRB conducts elections to determine the interest of employees in forming a union. It also investigates charges of unfair labor practice and prosecutes violations. Elections, investigations, and prosecution occur under the direction of the General Counsel's regional offices. Ajudication of violations and appeals is handled under the direction of the board.

negotiating committee Employees elected from within a designated bargaining unit to act as representatives of the employee organization in the development of a collective bargaining agreement; or a group of managers designated to represent management in labor negotiations.

nonstoppage strikes Procedures whereby labor and management mutually agree that work will not stop when the contract expires. To assure settlement, each side submits to penalties (usually financial) that pressure the negotiators to come to an agreement.

no raiding or nonraiding policies Agreements between affiliated unions of the AFL-CIO to respect each other's established collective bargaining relationships by not trying to organize workers already in some other AFL-CIO union. (These agreements are sometimes informally agreed to by unions not affiliated with the AFL-CIO.)

Norris-LaGuardia Act *See* Federal Anti-Injunction Act.

open shop An organization in which employees are free to join or not join a union as they see fit. *See also* union; closed shop.

personnel policies Statements governing the employer-employee relationship and its administration.

power The ability of one person (or group) to limit or expand the alternatives of another person (or group).

professional association A group or organization that exists to further the standards associated with a particular profession and/or provide continuing education for the members. *For groups that undertake collective action designed to improve wages, hours, or conditions of employment, see* union.

providers All individuals within the health care delivery system who contribute directly or indirectly to the process of providing health care; all employees and managers of a health care facility.

public sector Federal, state, county, and municipal governments and their subdivisions.

Railway Labor Act Federal law (1926) extending collective bargaining rights to interstate rail and air carriers and establishing the mechanism for its regulation.

Regional Director The official responsible for all operations (elections, investigations, and prosecution) within the geographical area covered by a given regional office of the General Counsel of the National Labor Relations Board.

right-to-work law A state law prohibiting agreements that require employees to be members or nonmembers of labor organizations.

security clause (maintenance of membership) A provision within the collective bargaining agreement which protects the status of the union by assuring some level of employee membership in the labor organization (e.g., a union shop clause).

steward A union official who helps employees to formalize and process grievances.

stipulated election An NLRB election held over the objections of one party (labor or, more commonly, management). The final outcome of a stipulated election is decided by the office of the General Counsel. *See also* consent election.

superseniority Seniority granted to certain groups of employees beyond that which length of service would justify. It is most commonly bestowed upon union officials to ensure that layoffs do not leave the employee group leaderless.

surprise strikes Strikes that take place with little or no notice given to management. Also called wildcat strikes.

Taft-Hartley Act *See* Labor Management Relations Act.

trilogy cases *See* Douglas doctrine.

trusteeship A process governed by the Landrum-Griffin Act whereby national or international unions can replace local union leaders for cause. A trusteeship of longer than eighteen months is presumed invalid.

unfair labor practice (ULP) Any action that interferes with the rights of employees or employers in violation of the National Labor Relations Act, as amended.

union shop An agreement whereby an employer may hire any employee but the new employee must join the union within a specified time period after being hired — usually thirty or sixty days. It also requires the employee to remain a member in good standing as a condition of retaining employment. Nonpayment of dues can lead to expulsion from the union and termination of employment.

union An organization having as one of its goals the improvement of wages, hours, and working conditions for its members. *For groups that exist solely to improve the image or standards of a profession, see* professional association.

wage reopener A clause within a contract which permits management or the union to reopen negotiations over wages to allow adjustments at stated intervals.

Wagner Act See National Labor Relations Act.

whipsawing A technique used by unions to secure favorable contracts. The union will use the contract obtained from one employer as the minimum acceptable goal in dealing with a second employer within the same industry. Gains from the second employer then become the minimum for dealing with a third employer, and so on.

wildcat strike A strike, usually conducted by a faction within the bargaining unit, that does not have the official consent of the union.

"yellow dog" contract An agreement (outlawed by the Norris-LaGuardia Act and made illegal by the National Labor Relations Act) whereby a worker signs an employment contract which requires the worker to refrain from joining a union.

The Labor Management Relations Act, 1947, as Amended by Public Laws 86-257, 1959,* and 93-360, 1974†‡

AN ACT

To amend the National Labor Relations Act, to provide additional facilities for the mediation of labor disputes affecting commerce, to equalize legal responsibilities of labor organizations and employers, and for other purposes.

Be it enacted by the Senate and House of Representatives of the United States of America in Congress assembled,

Short Title and Declaration of Policy

Section 1

(a) This Act may be cited as the "Labor Management Relations Act, 1947."

(b) Industrial strife which interferes with the normal flow of commerce

---

*Sec. 201(d) and (e) of the Labor-Management Reporting and Disclosure Act of 1959 which repealed Sec. 9(f), (g), and (h) of the Labor Management Relations Act, 1947, and Sec. 505 amending Sec. 302(a), (b), and (c) of the Labor Management Relations Act, 1947, took effect upon enactment of Public Law 86–257, Sept. 14, 1959. As to the other amendements of the Labor Management Relations Act, 1947, Sec. 707 of the Labor-Management Reporting and Disclosure Act provides:

The amendments made by this title shall take effect sixty days after the date of the enactment of this Act and no provision of this title shall be deemed to make an unfair labor practice, any act which is performed prior to such effective date which did not constitute an unfair labor practice prior thereto.

†The amendments to Secs. 2(2) and (14), 8(d) and (g), 19, and 213 became effective on the 30th day (Aug. 25, 1974) after its date of enactment, July 26, 1974.

‡For sale by the Superintendent of Documents, U.S. Government Printing Office, Washington, D.C. Price 45 cents. Stock No. 3100–00146.

and with the full production of articles and commodities for commerce, can be avoided or substantially minimized if employers, employees, and labor organizations each recognize under law one another's legitimate rights in their relations with each other, and above all recognize under law that neither party has any right in its relations with any other to engage in acts or practices which jeopardize the public health, safety, or interest.

It is the purpose and policy of this Act, in order to promote the full flow of commerce, to prescribe the legitimate rights of both employees and employers in their relations affecting commerce, to provide orderly and peaceful procedures for preventing the interference by either with the legitimate rights of the other, to protect the rights of individual employees in their relations with labor organizations whose activities affect commerce, to define and proscribe practices on the part of labor and management which affect commerce and are inimical to the general welfare, and to protect the rights of the public in connection with labor disputes affecting commerce.

TITLE I—AMENDMENT OF NATIONAL LABOR RELATIONS ACT

Section 101.

The National Labor Relations Act is hereby amended to read as follows:

Findings and Policies

Section 1

The denial by some employers of the right of employees to organize and the refusal by some employers to accept the procedure of collective bargaining lead to strikes and other forms of industrial strife or unrest, which have the intent or the necessary effect of burdening or obstructing commerce by (a) impairing the efficiency, safety, or operation of the instrumentalities of commerce; (b) occurring in the current of commerce; (c) materially affecting, restraining, or controlling the flow of raw materials or manufactured or processed goods from or into the channels of commerce, or the prices of such materials or goods in commerce; or (d) causing diminution of employment and wages in such volume as substantially to impair or disrupt the market for goods flowing from or into the channels of commerce.

The inequality of bargaining power between employees who do not possess full freedom of association or actual liberty of contract, and employers who are organized in the corporate or other forms of ownership association substantially burdens and affects the flow of commerce, and tends to aggravate recurrent business depressions, by depressing wage rates and the purchasing power of wage earners in industry and by preventing the stabilization of competitive wage rates and working conditions within and between industries.

Experience has proved that protection by law of the right of employees to organize and bargain collectively safeguards commerce from injury, impairment, or interruption, and promotes the flow of commerce by removing certain recognized sources of industrial strife and unrest, by encouraging practices fundamental to the friendly adjustment of industrial disputes arising out of differences as to wages, hours, or other working conditions, and by restoring equality of bargaining power between employers and employees.

Experience has further demonstrated that certain practices by some labor organizations, their officers, and members have the intent or the necessary effect of burdening or obstructing commerce by preventing the free flow of goods in such commerce through strikes and other forms of industrial unrest or through concerted activities which impair the interest of the public in the free flow of such commerce. The elimination of such practices is a necessary condition to the assurance of the rights herein guaranteed.

It is hereby declared to be the policy of the United States to eliminate the causes of certain substantial obstructions to the free flow of commerce and to mitigate and eliminate these obstructions when they have occurred by encouraging the practice and procedure of collective bargaining and by protecting the exercise by workers of full freedom of association, self-organization, and designation of representatives of their own choosing, for the purpose of negotiating the terms and conditions of their employment or other mutual aid or protection.

Definitions

Section 2
When used in this Act —
(1) The term "person" includes one or more individuals, labor organiza-

tions, partnerships, associations, corporations, legal representatives, trustees, trustees in bankruptcy, or receivers.

(2) The term "employer" includes any person acting as an agent of an employer, directly or indirectly, but shall not include the United States or any wholly owned Government corporation, or any Federal Reserve Bank, or any State or political subdivision thereof,* or any person subject to the Railway Labor Act, as amended from time to time, or any labor organization (other than when acting as an employer), or anyone acting in the capacity of officer or agent of such labor organization.

(3) The term "employee" shall include any employee, and shall not be limited to the employees of a particular employer, unless the Act explicitly states otherwise, and shall include any individual whose work has ceased as a consequence of, or in connection with, any current labor dispute or because of any unfair labor practice, and who has not obtained any other regular and substantially equivalent employment, but shall not include any individual employed as an agricultural laborer, or in the domestic service of any family or person at his home, or any individual employed by his parent or spouse, or any individual having the status of an independent contractor, or any individual employed as a supervisor, or any individual employed by an employer subject to the Railway Labor Act, as amended from time to time, or by any other person who is not an employer as herein defined.

(4) The term "representatives" includes any individual or labor organization.

(5) The term "labor organization" means any organization of any kind, or any agency or employee representation committee or plan, in which employees participate and which exists for the purpose, in whole or in part, of dealing with employers concerning grievances, labor disputes, wages, rates of pay, hours of employment, or conditions of work.

(6) The term "commerce" means trade, traffic, commerce, transporta‘ tion, or communication among the several States, or between the District of Columbia or any Territory of the United States and any State or other Territory, or between any foreign country and any State, Territory, or

---

*Pursuant to Public Law 93–360, 93d Cong., S. 3203, 88 Stat. 395, Sec. 2(2) is amended by deleting the phrase "or any corporation or association operating a hospital, if no part of the net earnings inures to the benefit of any private shareholder or individual,".

the District of Columbia, or within the District of Columbia or any Territory, or between points in the same State but through any other State or any Territory or the District of Columbia or any foreign country.

(7) The term "affecting commerce" means in commerce, or burdening or obstructing commerce or the free flow of commerce, or having led or tending to lead to a labor dispute burdening or obstructing commerce or the free flow of commerce.

(8) The term "unfair labor practice" means any unfair labor practice listed in section 8.

(9) The term "labor dispute" includes any controversy concerning terms, tenure or conditions of employment, or concerning the association or representation of persons in negotiating, fixing, maintaining, changing, or seeking to arrange terms or conditions of employment, regardless of whether the disputants stand in the proximate relation of employer and employee.

(10) The term "National Labor Relations Board" means the National Labor Relations Board provided for in section 3 of this Act.

(11) The term "supervisor" means any individual having authority, in the interest of the employer, to hire, transfer, suspend, lay off, recall, promote, discharge, assign, reward, or discipline other employees, or responsibly to direct them, or to adjust their grievances, or effectively to recommend such action, if in connection with the foregoing the exercise of such authority is not of a merely routine or clerical nature, but requires the use of independent judgment.

(12) The term "professional employee" means —

(a) any employee engaged in work (i) predominantly intellectual and varied in character as opposed to routine mental, manual, mechanical, or physical work; (ii) involving the consistent exercise of discretion and judgment in its performance; (iii) of such a character that the output produced or the result accomplished cannot be standardized in relation to a given period of time; (iv) requiring knowledge of an advanced type in a field of science or learning customarily acquired by a prolonged course of specialized intellectual instruction and study in an institution of higher learning or a hospital, as distinguished from a general academic education or from an apprenticeship or from training in the performance of routine mental, manual, or physical processes; or

(b) any employee, who (i) has completed the courses of specialized intellectual instruction and study described in clause (iv) of paragraph (a), and (ii) is performing related work under the supervision of a professional person to qualify himself to become a professional employee as defined in paragraph (a).

(13) In determining whether any person is acting as an "agent" of another person so as to make such other person responsible for his acts, the question of whether the specific acts performed were actually authorized or subsequently ratified shall not be controlling.

*(14) The term "health care institution" shall include any hospital, convalescent hospital, health maintenance organization, health clinic, nursing home, extended care facility, or other institution devoted to the care of sick, infirm, or aged person.

National Labor Relations Board

Section 3

(a) The National Labor Relations Board (hereinafter called the "Board") created by this Act prior to its amendment by the Labor Management Relations Act, 1947, is hereby continued as an agency of the United States, except that the Board shall consist of five instead of three members, appointed by the President by and with the advice and consent of the Senate. Of the two additional members so provided for, one shall be appointed for a term of five years and the other for a term of two years. Their successors, and the successors of the other members, shall be appointed for terms of five years each, excepting that any individual chosen to fill a vacancy shall be appointed only for the unexpired term of the member whom he shall succeed. The President shall designate one member to serve as Chairman of the Board. Any member of the Board may be removed by the President, upon notice and hearing, for neglect of duty or malfeasance in office, but for no other cause.

(b) The Board is authorized to delegate to any group of three or more members any or all of the powers which it may itself exercise. The Board is also authorized to delegate to its regional directors its powers under section 9 to determine the unit appropriate for the purpose of collective bargaining, to investigate and provide for hearings, and determine whether a question of representation exists, and to direct an election or take a secret ballot under subsection (c) or (e) of section 9 and certify the results thereof, except that upon the filing of a request therefor with the Board

*Pursuant to Public Law 93–360, 93d Cong., S. 3203, 88 Stat. 395, Sec. 2 is amended by adding subsection 14.

by any interested person, the Board may review any action of a regional director delegated to him under this paragraph, but such a review shall not, unless specifically ordered by the Board, operate as a stay of any action taken by the regional director. A vacancy in the Board shall not impair the right of the remaining members to exercise all of the powers of the Board, and three members of the Board shall, at all times, constitute a quorum of the Board, except that two members shall constitute a quorum of any group designated pursuant to the first sentence hereof. The Board shall have an official seal which shall be judicially noticed.

(c) The Board shall at the close of each fiscal year make a report in writing to Congress and to the President stating in detail the cases it has heard, the decisions it has rendered, the names, salaries, and duties of all employees and officers in the employ or under the supervision of the Board, and an account of all moneys it has disbursed.

(d) There shall be a General Counsel of the Board who shall be appointed by the President, by and with the advice and consent of the Senate, for a term of four years. The General Counsel of the Board shall exercise general supervision over all attorneys employed by the Board (other than trial examiners and legal assistants to Board members) and over the officers and employees in the regional offices. He shall have final authority, on behalf of the Board, in respect of the investigation of charges and issuance of complaints under section 10, and in respect of the prosecution of such complaints before the Board, and shall have such other duties as the Board may prescribe or as may be provided by law. In case of a vacancy in the office of the General Counsel the President is authorized to designate the officer or employee who shall act as General Counsel during such vacancy, but no person or persons so designated shall so act (1) for more than forty days when the Congress is in session unless a nomination to fill such vacancy shall have been submitted to the Senate, or (2) after the adjournment *sine die* of the session of the Senate in which such nomination was submitted.

Section 4

(a) Each member of the Board and the General Counsel of the Board shall receive a salary of $12,000* a year, shall be eligible for reappoint-

*Pursuant to Public Law 90–206, 90th Cong., 81 Stat. 644, approved Dec. 16, 1967, and in accordance with Sec. 225(f) (ii) thereof, effective in 1969, the salary of the Chairman of the Board shall be $40,000 per year and the salaries of the General Counsel and each Board member shall be $38,000 per year.

ment, and shall not engage in any other business, vocation, or employ-ment. The Board shall appoint an executive secretary, and such attorneys, examiners, and regional directors, and such other employees as it may from time to time find necessary for the proper performance of its duties. The Board may not employ any attorneys for the purpose of reviewing transcripts of hearings or preparing drafts of opinions except that any attorney employed for assignment as a legal assistant to any Board mem-ber may for such Board member review such transcripts and prepare such drafts. No trial examiner's report shall be reviewed, either before or after its publication, by any person other than a member of the Board or his legal assistant, and no trial examiner shall advise or consult with the Board with respect to exceptions taken to his findings, rulings, or recom-mendations. The Board may establish or utilize such regional, local, or other agencies, and utilize such voluntary and uncompensated services, as may from time to time be needed. Attorneys appointed under this section may, at the direction of the Board, appear for and represent the Board in any case in court. Nothing in this Act shall be construed to authorize the Board to appoint individuals for the purpose of conciliation or mediation, or for economic analysis.

(b) All of the expenses of the Board, including all necessary traveling and subsistence expenses outside the District of Columbia incurred by the members or employees of the Board under its orders, shall be allowed and paid on the presentation of itemized vouchers therefor approved by the Board or by any individual it designates for that purpose.

Section 5

The principal office of the Board shall be in the District of Columbia, but it may meet and exercise any or all of its powers at any other place. The Board may, by one or more of its members or by such agents or agencies as it may designate, prosecute any inquiry necessary to its func-tions in any part of the United States. A member who participates in such an inquiry shall not be disqualified from subsequently participating in a decision of the Board in the same case.

Section 6

The Board shall have authority from time to time to make, amend, and rescind, in the manner prescribed by the Administrative Procedure Act, such rules and regulations as may be necessary to carry out the provisions of this Act.

Rights of Employees

Section 7

Employees shall have the right to self-organization, to form, join, or assist labor organizations, to bargain collectively through representatives of their own choosing, and to engage in other concerted activities for the purpose of collective bargaining or other mutual aid or protection, and shall also have the right to refrain from any or all of such activities except to the extent that such right may be affected by an agreement requiring membership in a labor organization as a condition of employment as authorized in section 8(a)(3).

Unfair Labor Practices

Section 8

(a) It shall be an unfair labor practice for an employer —

(1) to interfere with, restrain, or coerce employees in the exercise of the rights guaranteed in section 7;

(2) to dominate or interfere with the formation or administration of any labor organization or contribute financial or other support to it: *Provided,* That subject to rules and regulations made and published by the Board pursuant to section 6, an employer shall not be prohibited from permitting employees to confer with him during working hours without loss of time or pay;

(3) by discrimination in regard to hire or tenure of employment or any term or condition of employment to encourage or discourage membership in any labor organization: *Provided,* That nothing in this Act, or in any other statute of the United States, shall preclude an employer from making an agreement with a labor organization (not established, maintained, or assisted by any action defined in section 8(a) of this Act as an unfair labor practice) to require as a condition of employment membership therein on or after the thirtieth day following the beginning of such employment or the effective date of such agreement, whichever is the later, (i) if such labor organization is the representative of the employees as provided in section 9(a), in the appropriate collective-bargaining unit covered by such agreement when made, and (ii) unless following an election held as provided in section 9(e) within one year preceding the effective date of such agreement, the Board shall have certified that at least a majority of the employees

eligible to vote in such election have voted to rescind the authority of such labor organization to make such an agreement: *Provided further,* That no employer shall justify any discrimination against an employee for nonmembership in a labor organization (A) if he has reasonable grounds for believing that such membership was not available to the employee on the same terms and conditions generally applicable to other members, or (B) if he has reasonable grounds for believing that membership was denied or terminated for reasons other than the failure of the employee to tender the periodic dues and the initiation fees uniformly required as a condition of acquiring or retaining membership;

(4) to discharge or otherwise discriminate against an employee because he has filed charges or given testimony under this Act;

(5) to refuse to bargain collectively with the representatives of his employees, subject to the provisions of section 9(a).

(b) It shall be an unfair labor practice for a labor organization or its agents —

(1) to restrain or coerce (A) employees in the exercise of the rights guaranteed in section 7: *Provided,* That this paragraph shall not impair the right of a labor organization to prescribe its own rules with respect to the acquisition or retention of membership therein; or (B) an employer in the selection of his representatives for the purposes of collective bargaining or the adjustment of grievances;

(2) to cause or attempt to cause an employer to discriminate against an employee in violation of subsection (a)(3) or to discriminate against an employee with respect to whom membership in such organization has been denied or terminated on some ground other than his failure to tender the periodic dues and the initiation fees uniformly required as a condition of acquiring or retaining membership;

(3) to refuse to bargain collectively with an employer, provided it is the representative of his employees subject to the provisions of section 9(a);

(4) (i) to engage in, or to induce or encourage any individual employed by any person engaged in commerce or in an industry affecting commerce to engage in, a strike or a refusal in the course of his employment to use, manufacture, process, transport, or otherwise handle or work on any goods, articles, materials, or commodities or to perform any services; or (ii) to threaten, coerce, or restrain any person engaged in commerce or in an industry affecting commerce, where in either case an object thereof is:

(A) forcing or requiring any employer or self-employed person to join any labor or employer organization or to enter into any agreement which is prohibited by section 8(e);

(B) forcing or requiring any person to cease using, selling, handling, transporting, or otherwise dealing in the products of any other producer, processor, or manufacturer, or to cease doing business with any other person, or forcing or requiring any other employer to recognize or bargain with a labor organization as the representative of his employees unless such labor organization has been certified as the representative of such employees under the provisions of section 9: *Provided,* That nothing contained in this clause (B) shall be construed to make unlawful, where not otherwise unlawful, any primary strike or primary picketing;

(C) forcing or requiring any employer to recognize or bargain with a particular labor organization as the representative of his employees if another labor organization has been certified as the representative of such employees under the provisions of section 9;

(D) forcing or requiring any employer to assign particular work to employees in a particular labor organization or in a particular trade, craft, or class rather than to employees in another labor organization or in another trade, craft, or class, unless such employer is failing to conform to an order or certification of the Board determining the bargaining representative for employees performing such work: *Provided,* That nothing contained in this subsection (b) shall be construed to make unlawful a refusal by any person to enter upon the premises of any employer (other than his own employer), if the employees of such employer are engaged in a strike ratified or approved by a representative of such employees whom such employer is required to recognize under this Act: *Provided further,* That for the purposes of this paragraph (4) only, nothing contained in such paragraph shall be construed to prohibit publicity, other than picketing, for the purpose of truthfully advising the public, including consumers and members of a labor organization, that a product or products are produced by an employer with whom the labor organization has a primary dispute and are distributed by another employer, as long as such publicity does not have an effect of inducing any individual employed by any person other than the primary employer in the course of his employment to refuse to pick up, deliver, or transport any goods, or not to perform any services, at the establishment of the employer engaged in such distribution;

(5) to require of employees covered by an agreement authorized under subsection (a)(3) the payment, as a condition precedent to becoming a member of such organization, of a fee in an amount which the Board finds excessive or discriminatory under all the circumstances. In making such a finding, the Board shall consider, among other relevant factors, the practices and customs of labor organizations in the particular industry, and the wages currently paid to the employees affected;

(6) to cause or attempt to cause an employer to pay or deliver or agree to pay or deliver any money or other thing of value, in the nature of an exaction, for services which are not performed or not to be performed; and

(7) to picket or cause to be picketed, or threaten to picket or cause to be picketed, any employer where an object thereof is forcing or requiring an employer to recognize or bargain with a labor organization as the representative of his employees, or forcing or requiring the employees of an employer to accept or select such labor organization as their collective bargaining representative, unless such labor organization is currently certified as the representative of such employees:

(A) where the employer has lawfully recognized in accordance with this Act any other labor organization and a question concerning representation may not appropriately be raised under section 9(c) of this Act,

(B) where within the preceding twelve months a valid election under section 9(c) of this Act has been conducted, or

(C) where such picketing has been conducted without a petition under section 9(c) being filed within a reasonable period of time not to exceed thirty days from the commencement of such picketing: *Provided,* That when such a petition has been filed the Board shall forthwith, without regard to the provisions of section 9(c)(1) or the absence of a showing of a substantial interest on the part of the labor organization, direct an election in such unit as the Board finds to be appropriate and shall certify the results thereof: *Provided further,* That nothing in this subparagraph (C) shall be construed to prohibit any picketing or other publicity for the purpose of truthfully advising the public (including consumers) that an employer does not employ members of, or have a contract with, a labor organization, unless an effect of such picketing is to induce any individual employed by any other person in the course of his employment, not to pick up, deliver or transport any goods or not to perform any services.

Nothing in this paragraph (7) shall be construed to permit any act which would otherwise be an unfair labor practice under this section 8(b).

(c) The expressing of any views, argument, or opinion, or the dissemination thereof, whether in written, printed, graphic, or visual form, shall not constitute or be evidence of an unfair labor practice under any of the provisions of this Act, if such expression contains no threat of reprisal or force or promise of benefit.

(d) For the purposes of this section, to bargain collectively is the performance of the mutual obligation of the employer and the representative of the employees to meet at reasonable times and confer in good faith with respect to wages, hours, and other terms and conditions of employment, or the negotiation of an agreement, or any question arising thereunder, and the execution of a written contract incorporating any agreement reached if requested by either party, but such obligation does not compel either party to agree to a proposal or require the making of a concession: *Provided,* That where there is in effect a collective-bargaining contract covering employees in an industry affecting commerce, the duty to bargain collectively shall also mean that no party to such contract shall terminate or modify such contract, unless the party desiring such termination or modification —

(1) serves a written notice upon the other party to the contract of the proposed termination or modification sixty days prior to the expiration date thereof, or in the event such contract contains no expiration date, sixty days prior to the time it is proposed to make such termination or modification;

(2) offers to meet and confer with the other party for the purpose of negotiating a new contract or a contract containing the proposed modifications;

(3) notifies the Federal Mediation and Conciliation Service within thirty days after such notice of the existence of a dispute, and simultaneously therewith notifies any State or Territorial agency established to mediate and conciliate disputes within the State or Territory where the dispute occurred, provided no agreement has been reached by that time; and

(4) continues in full force and effect, without resorting to strike or lockout, all the terms and conditions of the existing contract for a period of sixty days after such notice is given or until the expiration date of such contract, whichever occurs later:

The duties imposed upon employers, employees, and labor organizations by paragraphs (2), (3), and (4) shall become inapplicable upon an intervening certification of the Board, under which the labor organization or individual, which is a party to the contract, has been superseded as or ceased to be the representative of the employees subject to the provisions of section 9(a), and the duties so imposed shall not be construed as requiring either party to discuss or agree to any modification of the terms and conditions contained in a contract for a fixed period, if such modification is to become effective before such terms and conditions can be reopened under the provisions of the contract. Any employee who engages in a strike within *any notice period specified in this subsection*, or who engages in any strike within the appropriate period specified in subsection (g) of this section shall lose his status as an employee of the employer engaged in the particular labor dispute, for the purposes of sections 8, 9, and 10 of this Act, as amended, but such loss of status for such employee shall terminate if and when he is reemployed by such employer. *Whenever the collective bargaining involves employees of a health care institution, the provisions of this section 8(d) shall be modified as follows:

(A) The notice of section 8(d)(1) shall be ninety days; the notice of section 8(d)(3) shall be sixty days; and the contract period of section 8(d)(4) shall be ninety days;

(B) Where the bargaining is for an initial agreement following certification or recognition, at least thirty days' notice of the existence of a dispute shall be given by the labor organization to the agencies set forth in section 8(d)(3).

(C) After notice is given to the Federal Mediation and Conciliation Service under either clause (A) or (B) of this sentence, the Service shall promptly communicate with the parties and use its best efforts, by mediation and conciliation, to bring them to agreement. The parties shall participate fully and promptly in such meetings as may be undertaken by the Service for the purpose of aiding in a settlement of the dispute.

*Pursuant to Public Law 93–360, 93d Cong., S. 3203, 88 Stat. 396, the last sentence of Sec. 8(d) is amended by striking the words "the sixty day" and inserting the words "any notice" and by inserting before the words "shall lose" the phrase ", or who engages in any strike within the appropriate period specified in subsection (g) of this section." In addition, the end of paragraph Sec. 8(d) is amended by adding a new sentence "Whenever the collective bargaining . . . aiding in a settlement of the dispute."

(e) It shall be an unfair labor practice for any labor organization and any employer to enter into any contract or agreement, express or implied, whereby such employer ceases or refrains or agrees to cease or refrain from handling, using, selling, transporting or otherwise dealing in any of the products of any other employer, or to cease doing business with any other person, and any contract or agreement entered into heretofore or hereafter containing such an agreement shall be to such extent unenforceable and void: *Provided,* That nothing in this subsection (e) shall apply to an agreement between a labor organization and an employer in the construction industry relating to the contracting or subcontracting of work to be done at the site of the construction, alteration, painting, or repair of a building, structure, or other work: *Provided further,* That for the purposes of this subsection (e) and section 8(b)(4) (B) the terms "any employer", "any person engaged in commerce or in industry affecting commerce", and "any person" when used in relation to the terms "any other producer, processor, or manufacturer", "any other employer", or "any other person" shall not include persons in the relation of a jobber, manufacturer, contractor, or subcontractor working on the goods or premises of the jobber or manufacturer or performing parts of an integrated process of production in the apparel and clothing industry: *Provided further,* That nothing in this Act shall prohibit the enforcement of any agreement which is within the foregoing exception.

(f) It shall not be an unfair labor practice under subsections (a) and (b) of this section for an employer engaged primarily in the building and construction industry to make an agreement covering employees engaged (or who, upon their employment, will be engaged) in the building and construction industry with a labor organization of which building and construction employees are members (not established, maintained, or assisted by any action defined in section 8(a) of this Act as an unfair labor practice) because (1) the majority status of such labor organization has not been established under the provisions of section 9 of this Act prior to the making of such agreement, or (2) such agreement requires as a condition of employment, membership in such labor organization after the seventh day following the beginning of such employment or the effective date of the agreement, whichever is later, or (3) such agreement requires the employer to notify such labor organization of opportunities for employment with such employer, or gives such labor organization an opportunity to refer qualified applicants for such employment, or (4) such agreement specifies minimum training or experience qualifications for employment or provides for priority in opportunities for employment based upon length of service with such employer, in the industry or in the particular geographical area: *Provided,* That nothing in this subsection shall set aside the final proviso to section 8(a)(3) of this Act; *Provided further,* That any agreement which would be invalid, but for clause (1) of this subsection, shall not be a bar to a petition filed pursuant to section 9(c) or 9(e).*

†(g) A labor organization before engaging in any strike, picketing, or other concerted refusal to work at any health care institution shall, not less than ten days prior to such action, notify the institution in writing and the Federal Mediation and Conciliation Service of that intention, except that in the case of bargaining for an initial agreement following certification or recognition the notice required by this subsection shall not be given until the expiration of the period specified in clause (B) of the last sentence of section 8(d) of this Act. The notice shall state the date and time that such action will commence. The notice, once given, may be extended by the written agreement of both parties.

Representatives and Elections

Section 9

(a) Representatives designated or selected for the purposes of collective bargaining by the majority of the employees in a unit appropriate for such purposes, shall be the exclusive representatives of all the employees in such unit for the purposes of collective bargaining in respect to rates of pay, wages, hours of employment, or other conditions of employment: *Provided,* That any individual employee or a group of employees shall have the right at any time to present grievances to their employer and to have such grievances adjusted, without the intervention

---

*Sec. 8(f) is inserted in the Act by subsec. (a) of Sec. 705 of Public Law 86–257. Sec. 705(b) provides:

Nothing contained in the amendment made by subsection (a) shall be construed as authorizing the execution or application of agreements requiring membership in a labor organization as a condition of employment in any State of Territory in which such execution or application is prohibited by State or Territorial law.

†Pursuant to Public Law 93–360, 93d Cong., S. 3203, 88 Stat. 396, Sec. 8 is amended by adding subsection (g).

of the bargaining representative, as long as the adjustment is not inconsistent with the terms of a collective-bargaining contract or agreement then in effect: *Provided further,* That the bargaining representative has been given opportunity to be present at such adjustment.

(b) The Board shall decide in each case whether, in order to assure to employees the fullest freedom in exercising the rights guaranteed by this Act, the unit appropriate for the purposes of collective bargaining shall be the employer unit, craft unit, plant unit, or subdivision thereof: *Provided,* That the Board shall not (1) decide that any unit is appropriate for such purposes if such unit includes both professional employees and employees who are not professional employees unless a majority of such professional employees vote for inclusion in such unit; or (2) decide that any craft unit is inappropriate for such purposes on the ground that a different unit has been established by a prior Board determination, unless a majority of the employees in the proposed craft unit vote against separate representation or (3) decide that any unit is appropriate for such purposes if it includes, together with other employees, any individual employed as a guard to enforce against employees and other persons rules to protect property of the employer or to protect the safety of persons on the employer's premises; but no labor organization shall be certified as the representative of employees in a bargaining unit of guards if such organization admits to membership, or is affiliated directly or indirectly with an organization which admits to membership, employees other than guards.

(c) (1) Wherever a petition shall have been filed, in accordance with such regulations as may be prescribed by the Board—

(A) by an employee or group of employees or any individual or labor organization acting in their behalf alleging that a substantial number of employees (i) wish to be represented for collective bargaining and that their employer declines to recognize their representative as the representative defined in section 9(a), or (ii) assert that the individual or labor organization, which has been certified or is being currently recognized by their employer as the bargaining representative, is no longer a representative as defined in section 9(a); or

(B) by an employer, alleging that one or more individuals or labor organizations have presented to him a claim to be recognized as the representative defined in section 9(a);

the Board shall investigate such petition and if it has reasonable cause to believe that a question of representation affecting commerce exists shall provide for an appropriate hearing upon due notice. Such hearing may be conducted by an officer or employee of the regional office, who shall not make any recommendations with respect thereto. If the Board finds upon the record of such hearing that such a question of representation exists, it shall direct an election by secret ballot and shall certify the results thereof.

(2) In determining whether or not a question of representation affecting commerce exists, the same regulations and rules of decision shall apply irrespective of the identity of the persons filing the petition or the kind of relief sought and in no case shall the Board deny a labor organization a place on the ballot by reason of an order with respect to such labor organization or its predecessor not issued in conformity with section 10(c)

(3) No election shall be directed in any bargaining unit or any sub-division within which, in the preceding twelve-month period, a valid election shall have been held. Employees engaged in an economic strike who are not entitled to reinstatement shall be eligible to vote under such regulations as the Board shall find are consistent with the purposes and provisions of this Act in any election conducted within twelve months after the commencement of the strike. In any election where none of the choices on the ballot receives a majority, a run-off shall be conducted, the ballot providing for a selection between the two choices receiving the largest and second largest number of valid votes cast in the election.

(4) Nothing in this section shall be construed to prohibit the waiving of hearings by stipulation for the purpose of a consent election in conformity with regulations and rules of decision of the Board.

(5) In determining whether a unit is appropriate for the purposes specified in subsection (b) the extent to which the employees have organized shall not be controlling.

(d) Whenever an order of the Board made pursuant to section 10(c) is based in whole or in part upon facts certified following an investigation pursuant to subsection (c) of this section and there is a petition for the enforcement or review of such order, such certification and the record of such investigation shall be included in the transcript of the entire record required to be filed under section 10(e) or 10(f), and thereupon the decree of the court enforcing, modifying, or setting aside in whole or in part the order of the Board shall be made and entered upon the pleadings, testimony, and proceedings set forth in such transcript.

(e)(1) Upon the filing with the Board, by 30 per centum or more of the employees in a bargaining unit covered by an agreement between their employer and a labor organization made pursuant to section 8(a)(3), of a petition alleging they desire that such authority be rescinded, the Board shall take a secret ballot of the employees in such unit and certify the results thereof to such labor organization and to the employer.

(2) No election shall be conducted pursuant to this subsection in any bargaining unit or any subdivision within which, in the preceding twelve-month period, a valid election shall have been held.

Prevention of Unfair Labor Practices

Section 10

(a) The Board is empowered, as hereinafter provided, to prevent any person from engaging in any unfair labor practice (listed in section 8) affecting commerce. This power shall not be affected by any other means of adjustment or prevention that has been or may be established by agreement, law, or otherwise: *Provided,* That the Board is empowered by agreement with any agency of any State or Territory to cede to such agency jurisdiction over any cases in any industry (other than mining, manufacturing, communications, and transportation except where predominantly local in character) even though such cases may involve labor disputes affecting commerce, unless the provision of the State or Territorial statute applicable to the determination of such cases by such agency is inconsistent with the corresponding provision of this Act or has received a construction inconsistent therewith.

(b) Whenever it is charged that any person has engaged in or is engaging in any such unfair labor practice, the Board, or any agent or agency designated by the Board for such purposes, shall have power to issue and cause to be served upon such person a complaint stating the charges in that respect, and containing a notice of hearing before the Board or a member thereof, or before a designated agent or agency, at a place therein fixed, not less than five days after the serving of said complaint: *Provided,* That no complaint shall issue based upon any unfair labor practice occurring more than six months prior to the filing of the charge with the Board and the service of a copy thereof upon the person against whom such charge is made, unless the person aggrieved thereby was prevented from filing such charge by reason of service in the armed forces, in which event the six-month period shall be computed from the day of his discharge. Any such complaint may be amended by the member, agent, or agency conducting the hearing or the Board in its discretion at any time prior to the issuance of an order based thereon. The person so complained of shall have the right to file an answer to the original or amended complaint and to appear in person or otherwise and give testimony at the place and time fixed in the complaint. In the discretion of the member, agent, or agency conducting the hearing or the Board, any other person may be allowed to intervene in the said proceeding and to present testimony. Any such proceeding shall, so far as practicable, be conducted in accordance with the rules of evidence applicable in the district courts of the United States under the rules of civil procedure for the district courts of the United States, adopted by the Supreme Court of the United States pursuant to the Act of June 19, 1934 (U.S.C., title 28, secs. 723–B, 723–C).

(c) The testimony taken by such member, agent, or agency or the Board shall be reduced to writing and filed with the Board. Thereafter, in its discretion, the Board upon notice may take further testimony or hear argument. If upon the preponderance of the testimony taken the Board shall be of the opinion that any person named in the complaint has engaged in or is engaging in any such unfair labor practice, then the Board shall state its findings of fact and shall issue and cause to be served on such person an order requiring such person to cease and desist from such unfair labor practice, and to take such affirmative action including reinstatement of employees with or without back pay, as will effectuate the policies of this Act: *Provided,* That where an order directs reinstatement of an employee, back pay may be required of the employer or labor organization, as the case may be, responsible for the discrimination suffered by him: *And provided further,* That in determining whether a complaint shall issue alleging a violation of section 8(a)(1) or section 8(a)(2), and in deciding such cases, the same regulations and rules of decision shall apply irrespective of whether or not the labor organization affected is affiliated with a labor organization national or international in scope. Such order may further require such person to make reports from time to time showing the extent to which it has complied with the order. If upon the preponderance of the testimony taken the Board shall not be of the opinion that the person named in the complaint has engaged in or is engaging in any such unfair labor practice, then the Board shall state its findings of fact and shall issue an order dismissing the said complaint. No order of the Board shall require the reinstatement of any individual as an employee who has been suspended or discharged, or the payment to him of any back pay, if such individual was suspended or discharged for cause. In case the evidence is presented before a member of the Board, or before an examiner or examiners thereof, such member, or such examiner or examiners, as the case may be, shall issue and cause to be served on the parties to the proceeding a proposed report, together with a recommended order, which shall be filed with the Board, and if no exceptions are filed within twenty days after service thereof upon such parties, or within such further period as the Board may authorize, such recommended order shall become the order of the Board and become effective as therein prescribed.

(d) Until the record in a case shall have been filed in a court, as hereinafter provided, the Board may at any time, upon reasonable notice and in such manner as it shall deem proper, modify or set aside, in whole or in part, any finding or order made or issued by it.

(e) The Board shall have power to petition any court of appeals of the United States, or if all the courts of appeals to which application may be made are in vacation, any district court of the United States, within any circuit or district, respectively, wherein the unfair labor practice in question occurred or wherein such person resides or transacts business, for the enforcement of such order and for appropriate temporary relief or restraining order, and shall file in the court the record in the proceedings, as provided in section 2112 of title 28, United States Code. Upon the filing of such petition, the court shall cause notice thereof to be served upon such person, and thereupon shall have jurisdiction of the proceeding and of the question determined therein, and shall have power to grant such temporary relief or restraining order as it deems just and proper, and to make and enter a decree enforcing, modifying, and enforcing as so modified, or setting aside in whole or in part the order of the Board. No objection that has not been urged before the Board, its member, agent, or agency, shall be considered by the court, unless the failure or neglect to urge such objection shall be excused because of extraordinary circumstances. The findings of the Board with respect to questions of fact if supported by substantial evidence on the record considered as a whole shall be conclusive. If either party shall apply to the court for leave to adduce additional evidence and shall show to the satisfaction of the court that such additional evidence is material and that there were reasonable grounds for the failure to adduce such evidence in the hearing before the Board, its member, agent, or agency, the court may order such additional evidence to be taken before the Board, its member, agent, or agency, and to be made a part of the record. The Board may modify its findings as to the facts, or make new findings, by reason of additional evidence so taken and filed, and it shall file such modified or new findings, which findings with respect to questions of fact if supported by substantial evidence on the record considered as a whole shall be conclusive, and shall file its recommendations, if any, for the modification or setting aside of its original order. Upon the filing of the record with it the jurisdiction of the court shall be exclusive and its judgment and decree shall be final, except that the same shall be subject to review by the appropriate United States court of appeals if application was made to the district court as hereinabove provided, and by the Supreme Court of the United States upon writ of certiorari or certification as provided in section 1254 of title 28.

(f) Any person aggrieved by a final order of the Board granting or denying in whole or in part the relief sought may obtain a review of such order in any circuit court of appeals of the United States in the circuit wherein the unfair labor practice in question was alleged to have been engaged in or wherein such person resides or transacts business, or in the United States Court of Appeals for the District of Columbia, by filing in such court a written petition praying that the order of the Board be modified or set aside. A copy of such petition shall be forthwith transmitted by the clerk of the court to the Board, and thereupon the aggrieved party shall file in the court the record in the proceeding, certified by the Board, as provided in section 2112 of title 28, United States Code. Upon the filing of such petition, the court shall proceed in the same manner as in the case of an application by the Board under subsection (e) of this section, and shall have the same jurisdiction to grant to the Board such temporary relief or restraining order as it deems just and proper, and in like manner to make and enter a decree enforcing, modifying, and enforcing as so modified, or setting aside in whole or in part the order of the Board; the findings of the Board with respect to questions of fact if supported by substantial evidence on the record considered as a whole shall in like manner be conclusive.

(g) The commencement of proceedings under subsection (e) or (f) of this section shall not, unless specifically ordered by the court, operate as a stay of the Board's order.

(h) When granting appropriate temporary relief or a restraining order, or making and entering a decree enforcing, modifying, and enforcing as so modified, or setting aside in whole or in part an order of the Board, as provided in this section, the jurisdiction of courts sitting in equity shall not be limited by the Act entitled "An Act to amend the Judicial Code and to define and limit the jurisdiction of courts sitting in equity, and for other purposes," approved March 23, 1932 (U.S.C., Supp. VII, title 29, secs. 101–115).

(i) Petitions filed under this Act shall be heard expeditiously, and if possible within ten days after they have been docketed.

(j) The Board shall have power, upon issuance of a complaint as provided in subsection (b) charging that any person has engaged in or is engaging in an unfair labor practice, to petition any district court of the United States (including the District Court of the United States for the District of Columbia), within any district wherein the unfair labor practice in question is alleged to have occurred or wherein such person resides or transacts business, for appropriate temporary relief or restraining order. Upon the filing of any such petition the court shall cause notice thereof to be served upon such person, and thereupon shall have jurisdiction to grant to the Board such temporary relief or restraining order as it deems just and proper.

(k) Whenever it is charged that any person has engaged in an unfair labor practice within the meaning of paragraph (4)(D) of section 8(b), the Board is empowered and directed to hear and determine the dispute out of which such unfair labor practice shall have arisen, unless, within ten days after notice that such charge has been filed, the parties to such dispute submit to the Board satisfactory evidence that they have adjusted, or agreed upon methods for the voluntary adjustment of, the dispute. Upon compliance by the parties to the dispute with the decision of the Board or upon such voluntary adjustment of the dispute, such charge shall be dismissed.

(l) Whenever it is charged that any person has engaged in an unfair labor practice within the meaning of paragraph (4)(A), (B), or (C) of section 8(b), or section 8(e) or section 8(b)(7), the preliminary investigation of such charge shall be made forthwith and given priority over all other cases except cases of like character in the office where it is filed or to which it is referred. If, after such investigation, the officer or regional attorney to whom the matter may be referred has reasonable cause to believe such charge is true and that a complaint should issue, he shall, on behalf of the Board, petition any district court of the United States (including the District Court of the United States for the District of Columbia) within any district where the unfair labor practice in question has occurred, is alleged to have occurred, or wherein such person resides or transacts business, for appropriate injunctive relief pending the final adjudication of the Board with respect to such matter. Upon the filing of any such petition the district court shall have jurisdiction to grant such injunctive relief or temporary restraining order as it deems just and proper, notwithstanding any other provision of law: *Provided further,* That no temporary restraining order shall be issued without notice unless a petition alleges that substantial and irreparable injury to the charging party will be unavoidable and such temporary restraining order shall be effective for no longer than five days and will become void at the expiration of such period: *Provided further,* That such officer or regional attorney shall not apply for any restraining order under section 8(b)(7) if a charge against the employer under section 8(a)(2) has been filed and after the preliminary investigation, he has reasonable cause to believe that such charge is true and that a complaint should issue. Upon filing of any such petition the courts shall cause notice thereof to be served upon any person involved in the charge and such person, including the charging party, shall be given an opportunity to appear by counsel and present any relevant testimony: *Provided further,* That for the purposes of this subsection district courts shall be deemed to have jurisdiction of a labor organization (1) in the district in which such organization maintains its principal office, or (2) in any district in which its duly authorized officers or agents are engaged in promoting or protecting the interests of employee members. The service of legal process upon such officer or agent shall constitute service upon the labor organization and make such organizations a party to the suit. In situations where such relief is appropriate the procedure specified herein shall apply to charges with respect to section 8(b)(4)(D).

   (m) Whenever it is charged that any person has engaged in an unfair labor practice within the meaning of subsection (a)(3) or (b)(2) of section 8, such charge shall be given priority over all other cases except cases of like character in the office where it is filed or to which it is referred and cases given priority under subsection (1).

Investigatory Powers

Section 11

For the purpose of all hearings and investigations, which, in the opinion of the Board, are necessary and proper for the exercise of the powers vested in it by section 9 and section 10—

(1) The Board, or its duly authorized agents or agencies, shall at all reasonable times have access to, for the purpose of examination, and the right to copy any evidence of any person being investigated or proceeded against that relates to any matter under investigation or in question. The Board, or any member thereof, shall upon application of any party to such proceedings, forthwith issue to such party subpenas requiring the attendance and testimony of witnesses or the production of any evidence in such proceeding or investigation requested in such application. Within five days after the service of a subpena on any person requiring the production of any evidence in his possession or under his control, such person may petition the Board to revoke, and the Board shall revoke, such subpena if in its opinion the evidence whose production is required does not relate to any matter under investigation, or any matter in question in such proceedings, or if in its opinion such subpena does not describe with sufficient particularity the evidence whose production is required. Any member of the Board, or any agent or agency designated by the Board for such purposes, may administer oaths and affirmations, examine witnesses, and receive evidence. Such attendance of witnesses and the production of such evidence may be required from any place in the United States or any Territory or possession thereof, at any designated place of hearing.

(2) In case of contumacy or refusal to obey a subpena issued to any person, any district court of the United States or the United States courts of any Territory or possession, or the District Court of the United States for the District of Columbia, within the jurisdiction of which the inquiry is carried on or within the jurisdiction of which said person guilty of contumacy or refusal to obey is found or resides or transacts business, upon application by the Board shall have jurisdiction to issue to such person an order requiring such person to appear before the Board, its member, agent, or agency, there to produce evidence if so ordered, or there to give testimony touching the matter under investigation or in question; and any failure to obey such order of the court may be punished by said court as a contempt thereof.

(3)*

(4) Complaints, orders, and other process and papers of the Board, its member, agent, or agency, may be served either personally or by registered mail or by telegraph or by leaving a copy thereof at the principal office or place of business of the person required to be served. The verified return by the individual so serving the same setting forth the manner of such service shall be proof of the same, and the return post office receipt or telegraph receipt therefor when registered and mailed or telegraphed as aforesaid shall be proof of service of the same. Witnesses summoned before the Board, its member, agent, or agency, shall be paid the same fees and mileage that are paid witnesses in the courts of the United States, and witnesses whose depositions are taken and the persons taking the same shall severally be entitled to the same fees as are paid for like services in the courts of the United States.

(5) All process of any court to which application may be made under this Act may be served in the judicial district wherein the defendant or other person required to be served resides or may be found.

(6) The several departments and agencies of the Government, when directed by the President, shall furnish the Board, upon its request, all records, papers, and information in their possession relating to any matter before the Board.

Section 12

Any person who shall willfully resist, prevent, impede, or interfere with any member of the Board or any of its agents or agencies in the performance of duties pursuant to this Act shall be punished by a fine of not more than $5,000 or by imprisonment for not more than one year, or both.

Limitations

Section 13

Nothing in this Act, except as specifically provided for herein, shall be construed so as either to interfere with or impede or diminish in any way the right to strike, or to affect the limitations or qualifications on that right.

*Sec. 11(3) is repealed by Sec. 234, Public Law 91–452, 91st Cong., S. 30, 84 Stat. 926, Oct. 15, 1970. See Title 18, U.S.C. Sec. 6001, *et seq.*

Section 14

(a) Nothing herein shall prohibit any individual employed as a supervisor from becoming or remaining a member of a labor organization, but no employer subject to this Act shall be compelled to deem individuals defined herein as supervisors as employees for the purpose of any law, either national or local, relating to collective bargaining.

(b) Nothing in this Act shall be construed as authorizing the execution or application of agreements requiring membership in a labor organization as a condition of employment in any State or Territory in which such execution or application is prohibited by State or Territorial law.

(c)(1) The Board, in its discretion, may, by rule of decision or by published rules adopted pursuant to the Administrative Procedure Act, decline to assert jurisdiction over any labor dispute involving any class or category of employers, where, in the opinion of the Board, the effect of such labor dispute on commerce is not sufficiently substantial to warrant the exercise of its jurisdiction: *Provided,* That the Board shall not decline to assert jurisdiction over any labor dispute over which it would assert jurisdiction under the standards prevailing upon August 1, 1959.

(2) Nothing in this Act shall be deemed to prevent or bar any agency or the courts of any State or Territory (including the Commonwealth of Puerto Rico, Guam, and the Virgin Islands), from assuming and asserting jurisdiction over labor disputes over which the Board declines, pursuant to paragraph (1) of this subsection, to assert jurisdiction.

Section 15

Wherever the application of the provisions of section 272 of chapter 10 of the Act entitled "An Act to establish a uniform system of bankruptcy throughout the United States," approved July 1, 1898, and Acts amendatory thereof and supplementary thereto (U.S.C., title 11, sec. 672), conflicts with the application of the provisions of this Act, this Act shall prevail: *Provided,* That in any situation where the provisions of this Act cannot be validly enforced, the provisions of such other Acts shall remain in full force and effect.

Section 16

If any provision of this Act, or the application of such provision to any person or circumstances, shall be held invalid, the remainder of this Act, or the application of such provision to persons or circumstances other than those as to which it is held invalid, shall not be affected thereby.

Section 17
This Act may be cited as the "National Labor Relations Act."

Section 18
No petition entertained, no investigation made, no election held, and no certification issued by the National Labor Relations Board, under any of the provisions of section 9 of the National Labor Relations Act, as amended, shall be invalid by reason of the failure of the Congress of Industrial Organizations to have complied with the requirements of section 9(f), (g), or (h) of the aforesaid Act prior to December 22, 1949, or by reason of the failure of the American Federation of Labor to have complied with the provisions of section 9(f), (g), or (h) of the aforesaid Act prior to November 7, 1947: *Provided,* That no liability shall be imposed under any provision of this Act upon any person for failure to honor any election or certificate referred to above, prior to the effective date of this amendment: *Provided, however,* That this proviso shall not have the effect of setting aside or in any way affecting judgments or decrees heretofore entered under section 10(e) or (f) and which have become final.

Individuals with Religious Convictions

Section 19
Any employee of a health care institution who is a member of and adheres to established and traditional tenets or teachings of a bona fide religion, body, or sect which has historically held conscientious objections to joining or financially supporting labor organizations shall not be required to join or financially support any labor organization as a condition of employment; except that such employee may be required, in lieu of periodic dues and initiation fees, to pay sums equal to such dues and initiation fees to a nonreligious charitable fund exempt from taxation under section 501(c)(3) of the Internal Revenue Code, chosen by such employee from a list of at least three such funds, designated in a contract between such institution and a labor organization, or if the contract fails to designate such funds, then to any such fund chosen by the employee.

*Pursuant to Public Law 93–360, 93d Cong., S. 3203, 88 Stat. 397, the National Labor Relations Act is amended by adding Sec. 19.

Effective Date of Certain Changes*

Section 102

No provision of this title shall be deemed to make an unfair labor practice any act which was performed prior to the date of the enactment of this Act which did not constitute an unfair labor practice prior thereto, and the provisions of section 8(a)(3) and section 8(b)(2) of the National Labor Relations Act as amended by this title shall not make an unfair labor practice the performance of any obligation under a collective-bargaining agreement entered into prior to the date of the enactment of this Act, or (in the case of an agreement for a period of not more than one year) entered into on or after such date of enactment, but prior to the effective date of this title, if the performance of such obligation would not have constituted an unfair labor practice under section 8(3) of the National Labor Relations Act prior to the effective date of this title, unless such agreement was renewed or extended subsequent thereto.

Section 103

No provisions of this title shall affect any certification of representatives or any determination as to the appropriate collective-bargaining unit, which was made under section 9 of the National Labor Relations Act prior to the effective date of this title until one year after the date of such certification or if, in respect of any such certification, a collective-bargaining contract was entered into prior to the effective date of this title, until the end of the contract period or until one year after such date, whichever first occurs.

Section 104

The amendments made by this title shall take effect sixty days after the date of the enactment of this Act, except that the authority of the President to appoint certain officers conferred upon him by section 3 of the National Labor Relations Act as amended by this title may be exercised forthwith.

*The effective date referred to in Secs. 102, 103, and 104 is Aug. 22, 1947. For effective dates of 1959 and 1974 amendments, see footnotes on first page of this text.

TITLE II–CONCILIATION OF LABOR DISPUTES IN INDUSTRIES AFFECTING COMMERCE; NATIONAL EMERGENCIES

Section 201

That it is the policy of the United States that–

(a) sound and stable industrial peace and the advancement of the general welfare, health, and safety of the Nation and of the best interest of employers and employees can most satisfactorily be secured by the settlement of issues between employers and employees through the process of conference and collective bargaining between employers and the representatives of their employees;

(b) the settlement of issues between employers and employees through collective bargaining may be advanced by making available full and adequate governmental facilities for conciliation, mediation, and voluntary arbitration to aid and encourage employers and the representatives of their employees to reach and maintain agreements concerning rates of pay, hours, and working conditions, and to make all reasonable efforts to settle their differences by mutual agreement reached through conferences and collective bargaining or by such methods as may be provided for in any applicable agreement for the settlement of disputes; and

(c) certain controversies which arise between parties to collective-bargaining agreements may be avoided or minimized by making available full and adequate governmental facilities for furnishing assistance to employers and the representatives of their employees in formulating for inclusion within such agreements provision for adequate notice of any proposed changes in the terms of such agreements, for the final adjustment of grievances or questions regarding the application or interpretation of such agreements, and other provisions designed to prevent the subsequent arising of such controversies.

Section 202

(a) There is hereby created an independent agency to be known as the Federal Mediation and Conciliation Service (herein referred to as the "Service," except that for sixty days after the date of the enactment of this Act such term shall refer to the Conciliation Service of the Department of Labor). The Service shall be under the direction of a Federal Mediation and Conciliation Director (hereinafter referred to as the "Director"), who shall be appointed by the President by and with the advice and consent of the Senate.

The Director shall receive compensation at the rate of $12,000* per annum. The Director shall not engage in any other business, vocation, or employment.

(b) The Director is authorized, subject to the civil-service laws, to appoint such clerical and other personnel as may be necessary for the execution of the functions of the Service, and shall fix their compensation in accordance with the Classification Act of 1923, as amended, and may, without regard to the provisions of the civil-service laws and the Classification Act of 1923, as amended, appoint and fix the compensation of such conciliators and mediators as may be necessary to carry out the functions of the Service. The Director is authorized to make such expenditures for supplies, facilities, and services as he deems necessary. Such expenditures shall be allowed and paid upon presentation of itemized vouchers therefore approved by the Director or by any employee designated by him for that purpose.

(c) The principal office of the Service shall be in the District of Columbia, but the Director may establish regional offices convenient to localities in which labor controversies are likely to arise. The Director may by order, subject to revocation at any time, delegate any authority and discretion conferred upon him by this Act to any regional director, or other officer or employee of the Service. The Director may establish suitable procedures for cooperation with State and local mediation agencies. The Director shall make an annual report in writing to Congress at the end of the fiscal year.

(d) All mediation and conciliation functions of the Secretary of Labor or the United States Conciliation Service under section 8 of the Act entitled "An Act to create a Department of Labor," approved March 4, 1913 (U.S.C., title 29, sec. 51), and all functions of the United States Conciliation Service under any other law are hereby transferred to the Federal Mediation and Conciliation Service, together with the personnel and records of the United States Conciliation Service. Such transfer shall take effect upon the sixtieth day after the date of enactment of this Act. Such transfer shall not affect any proceedings pending before the United States Conciliation Service or any certification, order, rule, or regulation theretofore made by it or by the Secretary of Labor. The Director and the Service shall not be subject in any way to the jurisdiction or authority of the Secretary of labor or any official or division of the Department of Labor.

*Pursuant to Public Law 90–206, 90th Cong., 81 Stat. 644, approved Dec. 16, 1967, and in accordance with Sec. 225(f)(ii) thereof, effective in 1969, the salary of the Director shall be $40,000 per year.

Functions of the Service

Section 203

(a) It shall be the duty of the Service, in order to prevent or minimize interruptions of the free flow of commerce growing out of labor disputes, to assist parties to labor disputes in industries affecting commerce to settle such disputes through conciliation and mediation.

(b) The Service may proffer its services in any labor dispute in any industry affecting commerce, either upon its own motion or upon the request of one or more of the parties to the dispute, whenever in its judgment such dispute threatens to cause a substantial interruption of commerce. The Director and the Service are directed to avoid attempting to mediate disputes which would have only a minor effect on interstate commerce if State or other conciliation services are available to the parties. Whenever the Service does proffer its services in any dispute, it shall be the duty of the Service promptly to put itself in communication with the parties and to use its best efforts, by mediation and conciliation, to bring them to agreement.

(c) If the Director is not able to bring the parties to agreement by conciliation within a reasonable time, he shall seek to induce the parties voluntarily to seek other means of settling the dispute without resort to strike, lock-out, or other coercion, including submission to the employees in the bargaining unit of the employer's last offer of settlement for approval or rejection in a secret ballot. The failure or refusal of either party to agree to any procedure suggested by the Director shall not be deemed a violation of any duty or obligation imposed by this Act.

(d) Final adjustment by a method agreed upon by the parties is hereby declared to be the desirable method for settlement of grievance disputes arising over the application or interpretation of an existing collective-bargaining agreement. The Service is directed to make its conciliation and mediation services available in the settlement of such grievance disputes only as a last resort and in exceptional cases.

Section 204

(a) In order to prevent or minimize interruptions of the free flow of commerce growing out of labor disputes, employers and employees and their representatives, in any industry affecting commerce, shall—

(1) exert every reasonable effort to make and maintain agreements concerning rates of pay, hours, and working conditions, including

provision for adequate notice of any proposed change in the terms of such agreements;

(2) whenever a dispute arises over the terms or application of a collective-bargaining agreement and a conference is requested by a party or prospective party thereto, arrange promptly for such a conference to be held and endeavor in such conference to settle such dispute expeditiously; and

(3) in case such dispute is not settled by conference, participate fully and promptly in such meetings as may be undertaken by the Service under this Act for the purpose of aiding in a settlement of the dispute.

Section 205

(a) There is hereby created a National Labor-Management Panel which shall be composed of twelve members appointed by the President, six of whom shall be selected from among persons outstanding in the field of management and six of whom shall be selected from among persons outstanding in the field of labor. Each member shall hold office for a term of three years, except that any member appointed to fill a vacancy occurring prior to the expiration of the term for which his predecessor was appointed shall be appointed for the remainder of such term, and the terms of office of the members first taking office shall expire, as designated by the President at the time of appointment, four at the end of the first year, four at the end of the second year, and four at the end of the third year after the date of appointment. Members of the panel, when serving on business of the panel, shall be paid compensation at the rate of $25 per day, and shall also be entitled to receive an allowance for actual and necessary travel and subsistence expenses while so serving away from their places of residence.

(b) It shall be the duty of the panel, at the request of the Director, to advise in the avoidance of industrial controversies and the manner in which mediation and voluntary adjustment shall be administered, particularly with reference to controversies affecting the general welfare of the country.

National Emergencies

Section 206

Whenever in the opinion of the President of the United States, a threatened or actual strike or lock-out affecting an entire industry or a substantial part thereof engaged in trade, commerce, transportation, transmission, or communication among the several States or with foreign nations, or engaged in the production of goods for commerce, will, if permitted to occur or to continue, imperil the national health or safety, he may appoint a board of inquiry to inquire into the issues involved in the dispute and to make a written report to him within such time as he shall prescribe. Such report shall include a statement of the facts with respect to the dispute, including each party's statement of its position but shall not contain any recommendations. The President shall file a copy of such report with the Service and shall make its contents available to the public.

Section 207

(a) A board of inquiry shall be composed of a chairman and such other members as the President shall determine, and shall have power to sit and act in any place within the United States and to conduct such hearings either in public or in private, as it may deem necessary or proper, to ascertain the facts with respect to the causes and circumstances of the dispute.

(b) Members of a board of inquiry shall receive compensation at the rate of $50 for each day actually spent by them in the work of the board, together with necessary travel and subsistence expenses.

(c) For the purpose of any hearing or inquiry conducted by any board appointed under this title, the provisions of sections 9 and 10 (relating to the attendance of witnesses and the production of books, papers, and documents) of the Federal Trade Commission Act of September 16, 1914, as amended (U.S.C. 19, title 15, secs. 49 and 50, as amended), are hereby made applicable to the powers and duties of such board.

Section 208

(a) Upon receiving a report from a board of inquiry the President may direct the Attorney General to petition any district court of the United States having jurisdiction of the parties to enjoin such strike or lock-out or the continuing thereof, and if the court finds that such threatened or actual strike or lock-out—

(i) affects an entire industry or a substantial part thereof engaged in trade, commerce, transportation, transmission, or communication among the several States or with foreign nations, or engaged in the production of goods for commerce; and

(ii) if permitted to occur or to continue, will imperil the national health or safety, it shall have jurisdiction to enjoin any such strike or lock-out, or the continuing thereof, and to make such other orders as may be appropriate.

(b) In any case, the provisions of the Act of March 23, 1932, entitled "An Act to amend the Judicial Code and to define and limit the jurisdiction of courts sitting in equity, and for other purposes," shall not be applicable.

(c) The order or orders of the court shall be subject to review by the appropriate circuit court of appeals and by the Supreme Court upon writ of certiorari or certification as provided in sections 239 and 240 of the Judicial Code, as amended (U.S.C., title 29, secs. 346 and 347).

Section 209

(a) Whenever a district court has issued an order under section 208 enjoining acts or practices which imperil or threaten to imperil the national health or safety, it shall be the duty of the parties to the labor dispute giving rise to such order to make every effort to adjust and settle their differences, with the assistance of the Service created by this Act. Neither party shall be under any duty to accept, in whole or in part, any proposal of settlement made by the Service.

(b) Upon the issuance of such order, the President shall reconvene the board of inquiry which has previously reported with respect to the dispute. At the end of a sixty-day period (unless the dispute has been settled by that time), the board of inquiry shall report to the President the current position of the parties and the efforts which has been made for settlement, and shall include a statement by each party of its position and a statement of the employer's last offer of settlement. The President shall make such report available to the public. The National Labor Relations Board, within the succeeding fifteen days, shall take a secret ballot of the employees of each employer involved in the dispute on the question of whether they wish to accept the final offer of settlement made by their employer as stated by him and shall certify the results thereof to the Attorney General within five days thereafter.

Section 210

Upon the certification of the results of such ballot or upon a settlement being reached, whichever happens sooner, the Attorney General shall move the court to discharge the injunction, which motion shall then be granted and the injunction discharged. When such motion is granted, the President shall submit to the Congress a full and comprehensive report of the proceedings, including the findings of the board of inquiry and the ballot taken by the National Labor Relations Board, together with such recommendations as he may see fit to make for consideration and appropriate action.

Compilation of Collective-Bargaining Agreements, Etc.

Section 211

(a) For the guidance and information of interested representatives of employers, employees, and the general public, the Bureau of Labor Statistics of the Department of Labor shall maintain a file of copies of all available collective-bargaining agreements and other available agreements and actions thereunder settling or adjusting labor disputes. Such file shall be open to inspection under appropriate conditions prescribed by the Secretary of Labor, except that no specific information submitted in confidence shall be disclosed.

(b) The Bureau of Labor Statistics in the Department of Labor is authorized to furnish upon request of the Service, or employers, employees, or their representatives, all available data and factual information which may aid in the settlement of any labor dispute, except that no specific information submitted in confidence shall be disclosed.

Exemption of Railway Labor Act

Section 212

The provisions of this title shall not be applicable with respect to any matter which is subject to the provisions of the Railway Labor Act, as amended from time to time.

*Conciliation of Labor Disputes in the Health Care Industry

Section 213

(a) If, in the opinion of the Director of the Federal Mediation and

*Pursuant to Public Law 93–360, 93d Cong., S. 3203, 88 Stat. 396–397, Title II of the Labor Management Relations Act, 1947, is amended by adding Sec. 213.

Conciliation Service a threatened or actual strike or lockout affecting a health care institution will, if permitted to occur or to continue, substantially interrupt the delivery of health care in the locality concerned, the Director may further assist in the resolution of the impasse by establishing within 30 days after the notice to the Federal Mediation and Conciliation Service under clause (A) of the last sentence of section 8(d) (which is required by clause (3) of such section 8(d)), or within 10 days after the notice under clause (B), an impartial Board of Inquiry to investigate the issues involved in the dispute and to make a written report thereon to the parties within fifteen (15) days after the establishment of such a Board. The written report shall contain the findings of fact together with the Board's recommendations for settling the dispute, with the objective of achieving a prompt, peaceful and just settlement of the dispute. Each such Board shall be composed of such number of individuals as the Director may deem desirable. No member appointed under this section shall have any interest or involvement in the health care institutions or the employee organizations involved in the dispute.

(b) (1) Members of any board established under this section who are otherwise employed by the Federal Government shall serve without compensation but shall be reimbursed for travel, subsistence, and other necessary expenses incurred by them in carrying out its duties under this section.

(2) Members of any board established under this section who are not subject to paragraph (1) shall receive compensation at a rate prescribed by the Director but not to exceed the daily rate prescribed for GS-18 of the General Schedule under section 5332 of title 5, United States Code, including travel for each day they are engaged in the performance of their duties under this section and shall be entitled to reimbursement for travel, subsistence, and other necessary expenses incurred by them in carrying out their duties under this section.

(c) After the establishment of a board under subsection (a) of this section and for 15 days after any such board has issued its report, no change in the status quo in effect prior to the expiration of the contract in the case of negotiations for a contract renewal, or in effect prior to the time of the impasse in the case of an initial bargaining negotiation, except by agreement, shall be made by the parties to the controversy.

(d) There are authorized to be appropriated such sums as may be necessary to carry out the provisions of this section.

TITLE III

Suits by and Against Labor Organizations

Section 301

(a) Suits for violation of contracts between an employer and a labor organization representing employees in an industry affecting commerce as defined in this Act, or between any such labor organizations, may be brought in any district court of the United States having jurisdiction of the parties, without respect to the amount in controversy or without regard to the citizenship of the parties.

(b) Any labor organization which represents employees in an industry affecting commerce as defined in this Act and any employer whose activities affect commerce as defined in this Act shall be bound by the acts of its agents. Any such labor organization may sue or be sued as an entity and in behalf of the employees whom it represents in the courts of the United States. Any money judgment against a labor organization in a district court of the United States shall be enforceable only against the organization as an entity and against its assets, and shall not be enforceable against any individual member or his assets.

(c) For the purposes of actions and proceedings by or against labor organizations in the district courts of the United States, district courts shall be deemed to have jurisdiction of a labor organization (1) in the district in which such organization maintains its principal offices, or (2) in any district in which its duly authorized officers or agents are engaged in representing or acting for employee members.

(d) The service of summons, subpena, or other legal process of any court of the United States upon an officer or agent of a labor organization, in his capacity as such, shall constitute service upon the labor organization.

(e) For the purposes of this section, in determining whether any person is acting as an "agent" of another person so as to make such other person responsible for his acts, the question of whether the specific acts performed were actually authorized or subsequently ratified shall not be controlling.

Restrictions on Payments to Employee Representatives

Section 302

(a) It shall be unlawful for any employer or association of employers or any person who acts as a labor relations expert, adviser, or consultant to an employer or who acts in the interest of an employer to pay, lend, or deliver, or agree to pay, lend, or deliver, any money or other thing of value—

(1) to any representative of any of his employees who are employed in an industry affecting commerce; or

(2) to any labor organization, or any officer or employee thereof, which represents, seeks to represent, or would admit to membership, any of the employees of such employer who are employed in an industry affecting commerce; or

(3) to any employee or group or committee of employees of such employer employed in an industry affecting commerce in excess of their normal compensation for the purpose of causing such employee or group or committee directly or indirectly to influence any other employees in the exercise of the right to organize and bargain collectively through representatives of their own choosing; or

(4) to any officer or employee of a labor organization engaged in an industry affecting commerce with intent to influence him in respect to any of his actions, decisions, or duties as a representative of employees or as such officer or employee of such labor organization.

(b)(1) It shall be unlawful for any person to request, demand, receive, or accept, or agree to receive or accept, any payment, loan, or delivery of any money or other thing of value prohibited by subsection (a).

(2) It shall be unlawful for any labor organization, or for any person acting as an officer, agent, representative, or employee of such labor organization, to demand or accept from the operator of any motor vehicle (as defined in part II of the Interstate Commerce Act) employed in the transportation of property in commerce, or the employer of any such operator, any money or other thing of value payable to such organization or to an officer, agent, representative or employee thereof as a fee or charge for the unloading, or the connection with the unloading, of the cargo of such vehicle: *Provided,* That nothing in this paragraph shall be construed to make unlawful any payment by an employer to any of his employees as compensation for their services as employees.

(c) The provisions of this section shall not be applicable (1) in respect to any money or other thing of value payable by an employer to any of his employees whose established duties include acting openly for such employer in matters of labor relations or personnel administration or to any representative of his employees, or to any officer or employee of a labor organization, who is also an employee or former employee of such employer, as compensation for, or by reason of, his service as an employee of such employer; (2) with respect to the payment or delivery of any money or other thing of value in satisfaction of a judgment of any court or a decision or award of an arbitrator or impartial chairman or in compromise, adjustment, settlement, or release of any claim, complaint, grievance, or dispute in the absence of fraud or duress; (3) with respect to the sale or purchase of an article or commodity at the prevailing market price in the regular course of business; (4) with respect to money deducted from the wages of employees in payment of membership dues in a labor organization: *Provided,* That the employer has received from each employee, on whose account such deductions are made, a written assignment which shall not be irrevocable for a period of more than one year, or beyond the termination date of the applicable collective agreement, whichever occurs sooner; (5) with respect to money or other thing of value paid to a trust fund established by such representative, for the sole and exclusive benefit of the employees of such employer, and their families and dependents (or of such employees, families, and dependents jointly with the employees of other employers making similar payments, and their families and dependents): *Provided,* That (A) such payments are held in trust for the purpose of paying, either from principal or income or both, for the benefit of employees, their families and dependents, for medical or hospital care, pensions on retirement or death of employees, compensation for injuries or illness resulting from occupational activity or insurance to provide any of the foregoing, or unemployment benefits or life insurance, disability and sickness insurance, or accident insurance; (B) the detailed basis on which such payments are to be made is specified in a written agreement with the employer, and employees and employers are equally represented in the administration of such fund, together with such neutral persons as the representatives of the employers and the representatives of employees may agree upon and in the event the employer and employee groups deadlock on the administration of such fund and there are no neutral persons empowered to break such deadlock, such agreement provides that the two groups shall agree on an impartial umpire to decide such dispute, or in event of their failure to agree within a reasonable length of time, an impartial umpire to decide such dispute shall, on petition of either group, be appointed by the district court of the United States for the district where the trust fund

has its principal office, and shall also contain provisions for an annual
audit of the trust fund, a statement of the results of which shall be available for inspection by interested persons at the principal office of the
trust fund and at such other places as may be designated in such written
agreement; and (C) such payments as are intended to be used for the
purpose of providing pensions or annuities for employees are made to a
separate trust which provides that the funds held therein cannot be used
for any purpose other than paying such pensions or annuities; (6) with
respect to money or other thing of value paid by any employer to a trust
fund established by such representative for the purpose of pooled vacation,
holiday, severance or similar benefits, or defraying costs of apprenticeship
or other training program; *Provided,* That the requirements of clause (B)
of the proviso to clause (5) of this subsection shall apply to such trust
funds; or (7) with respect to money or other thing of value paid by any
employer to a pooled or individual trust fund established by such representative for the purpose of (A) scholarships for the benefit of employees,
their families, and dependents for study at educational institutions, or
(B) child care centers for preschool and school age dependents of employees: *Provided,* That no labor organization or employer shall be required to bargain on the establishment of any such trust fund, and refusal
to do so shall not constitute an unfair labor practice: *Provided further,*
That the requirements of clause (B) of the proviso to clause (5) of this
subsection shall apply to such trust funds*; or (8) with respect to money
or any other thing of value paid by any employer to a trust fund established by such representative for the purpose of defraying the costs of
legal services for employees, their families, and dependents for counsel
or plan of their choice: *Provided,* That the requirements of clause (B)
of the proviso to clause (5) of this subsection shall apply to such trust
funds: *Provided further,* That no such legal services shall be furnished;
(A) to initiate any proceeding directed (i) against any such employer or
its officers or agents except in workman's compensation cases, or (ii) against
such labor organization, or its parent or subordinate bodies, or their
officers or agents, or (iii) against any other employer or labor organization, or their officers or agents, in any matter arising under the National

*Sec. 302(c)(7) has been added by Public Law 91–86, 91st Cong., S. 2068,
83 Stat. 133, approved Oct. 14, 1969; Sec. 302(c)(8) was added by Public Law
93–95, 93d Cong., S. 1423, 87 Stat. 314–315, approved Aug. 15, 1973.

Labor Relations Act, as amended, or this Act; and (B) in any proceeding where a labor organization would be prohibited from defraying the costs of legal services by the provisions of the Labor-Management Reporting and Disclosure Act of 1959.

(d) Any person who willfully violates any of the provisions of this section shall, upon conviction thereof, be guilty of a misdemeanor and be subject to a fine of not more than $10,000 or to imprisonment for not more than one year, or both.

(e) The district courts of the United States and the United States courts of the Territories and possessions shall have jurisdiction, for cause shown, and subject to the provisions of section 17 (relating to notice to opposite party) of the Act entitled "An Act to supplement existing laws against unlawful restraints and monopolies, and for other purposes," approved October 15, 1914, as amended (U.S.C., title 28, sec. 381), to restrain violations of this section, without regard to the provisions of sections 6 and 20 of such Act of October 15, 1914, as amended (U.S.C., title 15, sec. 17, and title 29, sec. 52), and the provisions of the Act entitled "An Act to amend the Judicial Code and to define and limit the jurisdiction of courts sitting in equity, and for other purposes," approved March 24, 1932 (U.S.C., title 29, secs. 101—115).

(f) This section shall not apply to any contract in force on the date of enactment of this Act, until the expiration of such contract, or until July 1, 1948, whichever first occurs.

(g) Compliance with the restrictions contained in subsection (c)(5)(B) upon contributions to trust funds, otherwise lawful, shall not be applicable to contributions to such trust funds established by collective agreement prior to January 1, 1946, nor shall subsection (c)(5)(A) be construed as prohibiting contributions to such trust funds if prior to January 1, 1947, such funds contained provisions for pooled vacation benefits.

Boycotts and Other Unlawful Combinations

Section 303

(a) It shall be unlawful, for the purpose of this section only, in an industry or activity affecting commerce, for any labor organization to engage in any activity or conduct defined as an unfair labor practice in section 8(b)(4) of the National Labor Relations Act, as amended.

(b) Whoever shall be injured in his business or property by reason of

any violation of subsection (a) may sue therefore in any district court
of the United States subject to the limitations and provisions of section
301 hereof without respect to the amount in controversy, or in any other
court having jurisdiction of the parties, and shall recover the damages by
him sustained and the cost of the suit.

Restriction on Political Contributions

Section 304

Section 313 of the Federal Corrupt Practices Act, 1925 (U.S.C., 1940
edition, title 2, sec. 251; Supp. V, title 50, App. sec. 1509), as amended,
is amended to read as follows:

Section 313

It is unlawful for any national bank, or any corporation organized by
authority of any law of Congress to make a contribution or expenditure
in connection with any election to any political office, or in connection
with any primary election or political convention or caucus held to select
candidates for any political office, or for any corporation whatever, or
any labor organization to make a contribution or expenditure in connection with any election at which Presidential and Vice Presidential
electors or a Senator or Representative in, or a Delegate or Resident
Commissioner to Congress are to be voted for, or in connection with any
primary election or political convention or caucus held to select candidates for any of the foregoing offices, or for any candidate, political
committee, or other person to accept or receive any contribution prohibited by this section. Every corporation or labor organization which
makes any contribution or expenditure in violation of this section shall
be fined not more than $5,000; and every officer or director of any
corporation, or officer of any labor organization, who consents to any
contribution or expenditure by the corporation or labor organization,
as the case may be, in violation of this section shall be fined not more than
$1,000 or imprisoned for not more than one year, or both. For the
purposes of this section "labor organization" means any organization of
any kind, or any agency or employee representation committee or plan,
in which employees participate and which exists for the purpose, in whole
or in part, of dealing with employers concerning grievances, labor disputes,
wages, rates of pay, hours of employment, or conditions of work.

TITLE IV

Creation of Joint Committee to Study and Report on Basic Problems Affecting Friendly Labor Relations and Productivity

TITLE V

Definitions

Section 501

When used in this Act—

(1) The term "industry affecting commerce" means any industry or activity in commerce or in which a labor dispute would burden or obstruct commerce or tend to burden or obstruct commerce or the free flow of commerce.

(2) The term "strike" includes any strike or other concerted stoppage of work by employees (including a stoppage by reason of the expiration of a collective-bargaining agreement) and any concerted slow-down or other concerted interruption of operations by employees.

(3) The terms "commerce," "labor disputes," "employer," "employee," "labor organization," "representative," "person," and "supervisor" shall have the same meaning as when used in the National Labor Relations Act as amended by this Act.

Saving Provision

Section 502

Nothing in this Act shall be construed to require an individual employee to render labor or service without his consent, nor shall anything in this Act be construed to make the quitting of his labor by an individual employee an illegal act; nor shall any court issue any process to compel the performance by an individual employee of such labor or service, without his consent; nor shall the quitting of labor by an employee or employees in good faith because of abnormally dangerous conditions for work at the place of employment of such employee or employees be deemed a strike under this Act.

Separability

Section 503

If any provision of this Act, or the application of such provision to any person or circumstance, shall be held invalid, the remainder of this Act, or the application of such provision to persons or circumstances other than those as to which it is held invalid, shall not be affected thereby.

reasons for nonmembership in
unions, 33–34, 38–39,
80–81
reasons for union membership,
31–33, 36–37
responsibilities of, 8–9, 38–39
rights of, 8, 35, 36–37, 47–48.
See also Labor-Manage-
ment Reporting and
Disclosure Act (1959),
Title I
types of, 79
Nonprofit Health Care Amendments to Labor Manage-
ment Relations Act, 78
Nonstoppage strikes, 152–153
Norris-LaGuardia Act (1932), 148
No-strike laws, 47
Nurses, 175
changes in role of, 2, 4–5
graduate, 80
registered, 80
Nursing homes, 58, 130

Occupational Safety and Health
Act, union lobbying for,
17, 45, 54
Organizing. *See* Union organizing
Overtime, 108

Part-time employees, 81
Paternalistic management, 33
Personnel directors, 95
Personnel policies, 167–168, 176
Peter Principle, 92
Petitions, antiunion, 49
Philosophy of labor relations,
170–171
Picketing, 59–61, 76
informational, 59–60, 61
recognition, 60–61
Power
abuse of, 9
of administrators. *See* Adminis-
trators, power of
balance of, 1, 36

importance of, 9
benefits of, 37
of clients. *See* Clients
equalization of, 36
external sources of. *See* Clients;
Government, regulation of
health care industry
of government. *See* Government,
regulation of health care
industry
historical development of, 3–8
imbalances, repercussions of,
9–10
influence of education and skill
on, 2, 4–5
interdependence and, 9–10
in negotiations, 54
of nonadministrative personnel.
See Nonadministrative
personnel, power of
of providers. *See* Administrators,
power of; Nonadministra-
tive personnel, power of
regulation of. *See* Government,
regulation of health care
industry
relationships, changes in, 107
of solidarity, 36
sources of, 1–3
Precedents, 161–163, 166–167
Prentice-Hall, Inc., publications
on labor law, 55
Productivity of workers, 53
Professional associations. *See also*
Unions
conflicts with unions, 40, 41,
179
defined, 14
dilemma of, 9, 14
election of officers, 23
exclusion from, 9
organizational structure, 22–23
divisions of, 22
local districts and councils, 22
national association, 22–23
professional division, 22

initial contracts, 145
protection of, by NLRB, 147
reason for nonmembership in
  unions, 34
types of
  economic, 145–146
  illegal, 57–60
  sit-down, 147
  surprise, 117
  sympathy, 147
  unfair labor practice, 146
underutilization of facilities
  due to, 10
Strikers, 143, 147–148
National Labor Relations
  Board's protection of, 143
Supervisors, 80, 92, 115, 177,
186. *See also* Administrators
Surveillance of union members, 52
Sweetheart arrangements, 162

Taft-Hartley Act. *See* Labor
  Management Relations
  Act (1947)
Tax laws, 183
Technical employees, 79
Technocrats, 4–5
Temporary employees, 81
Temporary restraining order, 148.
  See also Injunctions
Training in labor relations, 169
Trilogy, 138
Truman, Harry, 7n
Trustee provisions, 94. *See also*
  Labor-Management Re-
  porting and Disclosure
  Act (1959)
Turnover, employee, 91, 178

Unfair labor practices, 48. *See
  also* Labor Management
  Relations Act (1947)
Union activity, knowledge of by
  employer, 52
Union constitution, 23, 94

Union contract. *See* Labor-
  management contract
Union corruption, 165
Union members
  Bill of Rights, 23–27. *See also*
    Labor-Management Re-
    porting and Disclosure
    Act (1959), Title I
  questioning of, 52, 55
  survival needs of, 160–161
Union negotiations. *See*
  Negotiations
Union officials
  national president, role of, 17
  national representative, role of,
    16, 17
  national secretary-treasurer,
    role of, 18
  stewards, role of, 16, 129, 131, 160
  survival needs of, 160–161
Union organizer, role of, 98,
  100–101
Union organizing, 87–103, 158,
  167–168
  accuracy of information, 95
  assumptions by administrators,
    88–89
  assumptions by organizers, 89
  centralization of information,
    96–97
  centralization of responsibility,
    97
  comparative analysis, 95
  contract administration, rela-
    tionship to, 89–90
  contract negotiations, relation-
    ship to, 89–90
  factors leading to, 90–92
  free speech during, 96
  get-out-the-vote committees, 101
  good faith doubt of union
    majority, 100–101
  indications of, 92–94
  in-house organizing committee,
    99
  initial meeting, 99

United Farm Workers, 58
United States Supreme Court,
148, 176

Wages, 183–184
Wagner Act, 6–7
Women
    attitudes toward unions, 34
    leadership by, 41

Work-place rules, 15, 35, 53
Work practices, restrictions on, 3,
    5, 38
Working conditions, 53

Yellow-dog contracts, 48

Zero-sum relationship, 157